the

energy

plan

the energy plan

tap your inner resource

for maximum vitality

Aliza Baron Cohen

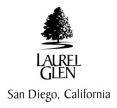

LAUREL GLEN

San Diego, California

Laurel Glen Publishing
An imprint of the Advantage Publishers Group
5880 Oberlin Drive, San Diego, CA 92121-4794
www.laurelglenbooks.com

First published in Great Britain in 2002 by Kyle Cathie Ltd.

Text © Aliza Baron Cohen, 2002
Design and layout © Mark Buckingham, 2002
Special photography © Tim Winter except for those images listed on page 223
Illustrations on pages 33 and 69 © David West

All notations of errors or omissions should be addressed to Laurel Glen Publishing, editorial
department, at the above address. All other correspondence (author inquiries, permissions, and rights)
concerning the content of this book should be addressed to Kyle Cathie Ltd, 122 Arlington Road,
London NW1 7HP, England.

ISBN 1-57145-846-8
Library of Congress Cataloging-in-Publication Data available upon request.

Color separation by Sang Choy International
Printed in Singapore by Kyodo Printing Co.

1 2 3 4 5   06 05 04 03 02

Contents

Chapter 1 What is energy? ———————————— 10

Chapter 2 Increase your energy ——————————— 28

Chapter 3 Energy plans ——————————— 158

Chapter 4 Energy for life ——————————— 200

Foreword

Pete Cohen, Life Strategist, author, and health and fitness professional

Energy is something that we all talk about and desire in our lives. Everyone has been in a position in their life where they have craved more energy—the energy to concentrate, the energy to get well, the energy to stay awake, the energy that enables us to be healthy and live a long life.

But what exactly is energy and where do you get it from? The mere mention of the word to some people makes them uncomfortable, as it calls to mind connotations of mysticism or spirituality.

We really do not know that much when it comes to understanding how the human mind and body work. We are made up of over 10 billion cells and modern science only knows and understands about 5 percent of how we work.

Conventional medicine has been slow to catch on to some of the principles that have existed for thousands of years in other cultures. For example, the manifestation of energy and its flow through the body is the foundation of Chinese medicine. Conventional medicine is based on scientific understanding and proof of how things work.

I once heard about a research project on acupuncture. The study wanted to scientifically prove how it works, exploring the body's meridians and energy points. When I heard about this and the huge amount of money that had gone into it I thought how much more useful the study would have been if it had simply researched acupuncture's effectiveness as a treatment by giving it to people and monitoring their progress.

This book will guide you through a transformation process in which you begin to experience a deeper and more practical understanding of energy. By following the practical and simple exercises you will learn to manifest more energy than you ever thought possible.

My philosophy in life is: if something works for you, then do it. This book will show you many simple but highly effective techniques and exercises that will really work to increase your energy.

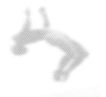

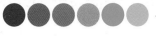
Introduction

Do you wake up every morning wondering how you will find enough energy to get through the day?

Do you sometimes feel as though you've been tired for years and can't even remember when you last had any energy? Does it often seem to you that everyone else copes with the day-to-day hustle and bustle of life only too well, while you plod along at your own slow pace? Or perhaps you just find yourself sometimes wishing for a little more energy to allow you to take on a new hobby or activity?

If so, this book is for you, and for millions of others like you. Believe it or not, tiredness and lack of energy affect us all at one time or another, and in spite of outward appearances, there are very few of us who actually live life at an optimum energy level.

Of course, in some cases an underlying health problem may be causing feelings of tiredness and lethargy, and if you suspect that this is the case (see pages 24–25), it is essential for you to see your physician for a thorough checkup.

In addition, *The Energy Plan* looks at pregnancy and early parenthood, and why some people find themselves exhausted and barely able to cope after having a baby, while others in similar situations seem to glow with energy. Having had a baby myself a year ago, I know only too well how energy can dip during these times. The book

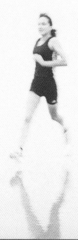

offers advice on how to take care of yourself during emotionally or physically demanding times, and how to conserve and build your energy when you most need it. There is a section for older people (written by my own mother, a vibrant woman and mother of five), and general information on therapies, diet, and exercise, as

However, other factors such as late nights, stress at work or at home, or jet lag from traveling, can all conspire to make us function and feel below par some, or all, of the time.

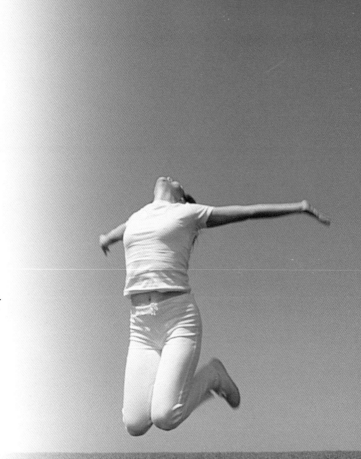

well as specific plans to follow.

This book is designed to help you regardless of your age or current physical condition. It's about quality of life and how to improve it by giving you the energy and zest for life that you deserve.

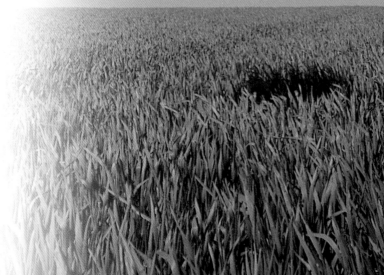

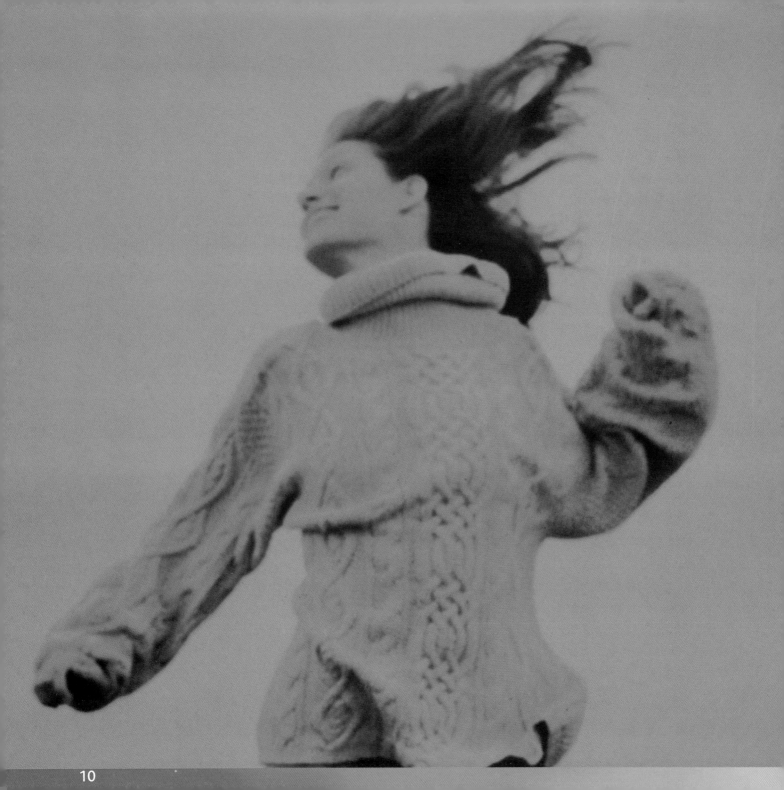

CHAPTER 1
What is energy?

In the West we tend to see energy in terms of how much we are able to do.

From an early age we are taught that energy in (e.g., food) = energy out (e.g., being able to work hard and play hard). We take energy in through food and air, process it, and pass it out again. The amount of energy we have depends then on our eating well, breathing correctly, and not allowing ourselves to become overworked or stressed.

Imagine your energy levels as a bank account. If you keep taking energy out without putting something back in, you will start to use up your savings/reserves. Therefore, in order to achieve optimum energy levels, it is vital that we learn how to replenish our savings/reserves through, for example, meditation, good diet, and so on. We must also develop an awareness of our own energy levels so we know when we are overdoing it, and take the opportunity to recharge our batteries.

Ancient civilizations believed that our bodies are made up not only of skin, muscle, and bone, but of an energy that cannot be seen even under a microscope. Most cultures and traditions see energy as the essence of life or our life force: the Chinese call it *qi*, the Japanese call it *ki*, the Indians call it *prana*, and in some parts of the Middle East it is known as *quwa*. Whatever it is called, healers from all these different cultures work with energy centers and pathways. Shamans use rituals and ceremonies to shift energies. Eastern traditions also believe in disciplines such as t'ai chi, qi gong, and yoga to help stimulate energy flow. Clairvoyants and psychics also work with energy stemming from an aura that surrounds the body, which they describe as many colors of light.

Ultimately, it does not really matter how you view energy, because it is always the same thing but viewed from different cultural perspectives. When someone feels they are lacking in energy, it can mean one of two things: Either there is a blockage preventing the free flow of energy (caused by factors such as stress, emotional or physical trauma, smoking, and alcohol and drug abuse), or there was never enough energy in the first place. Imagine your body's energy as water in a river: If nothing is in its way, the water can flow freely, but if there is an obstruction, it will become stagnant. Equally, if there is not enough water in the river, it will dry up altogether. It is vital then to find ways to build up our energy supply while also making efforts to continually stimulate and balance its natural flow.

In order to better understand the underlying principles behind many of the exercises that will be used later in the book—such as qi gong and yoga—let's take a look at their meanings, and their relevance, when trying to work on our energy levels.

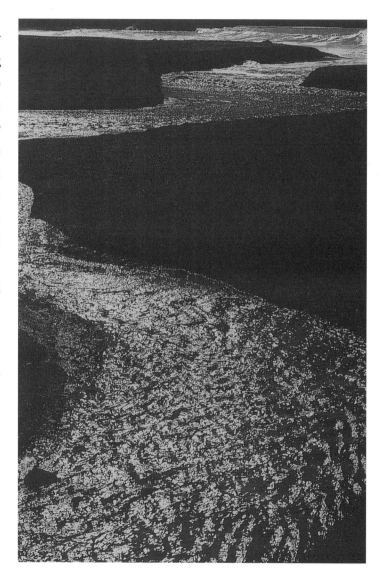

Qi

Qi is a key concept in traditional Chinese medicine, similar to prana in Indian philosophy (see p. 14) and ki in Japanese. Chinese medicine views the mind and body working due to the interaction of vital substances. They see the body and mind as energy (our get-up-and-go energy) and vital energy (the energy needed for all our systems to function) interacting together to make a person. At the basis of all of this is qi. All the other vital substances, such as blood, body fluids, *shen* (mind), etc., are all also qi manifested in different forms.

The Chinese believe that inner harmony is dependent upon a healthy, balanced, and unobstructed flow of qi. A smooth, uninterrupted flow will mean that you relax easily; feel energetic, happy, and are able to cope with difficult situations; sleep well and wake up rejuvenated; and have the ability to fight off disease with an efficient immune system.

Acupuncturists work with the qi that moves through the meridians, or channels, of the body. Qi is also used in the practice of feng shui, where the energy of a house may be studied and furniture and other objects placed in certain positions to improve the flow of qi.

Qi then is a vital essence found in all things. It is the force that drives every cell of our bodies, without which we would die.

Qi supports, nourishes, and defends us against mental, emotional, and physical problems. It is an invisible electromagnetic force that modern research in the West interprets as energy.

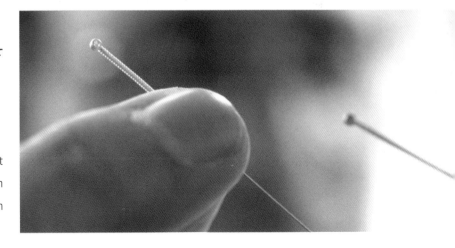

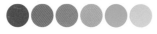

Prana

Prana is a Sanskrit word for the energy that sustains all life and creation.

It is thought to be all the energy that exists in the universe, and strength, power, vitality, life, and spirit are all forms of prana. It is used in Indian medicine and the practice of yoga. Ayurvedic medicine (the ancient system of medicine practiced in India) also talks of prana, using it to denote the living energy that fills our food, bodies, and all our relationships.

The philosophy of energy While many ancient philosophies consider the concept of universal energy, it also plays a part in modern philosophies such as quantum physics, which holds that everything that exists in the universe is made up of patterns of energy (for example, atoms). Like atoms, people and objects are made up of groups of vibrating energetic particles (also known as prana/qi).

Indian philosophy and medicine teaches that we take prana into our bodies through the *nadis*.

These are subtle energy channels that feed our *chakras*. Nadis are very similar to the subtle energy channels/meridians in Chinese medicine, and as in that discipline, it is important to make sure prana flows smoothly. Yoga postures, a healthy diet, sunlight, fresh air, meditation, and correct breathing techniques can all encourage this.

Yoga practitioners believe and teach that by using yoga techniques, prana can be controlled, directed, and stored at will, and that by learning to tap into it, you can acquire endless energy. Some of these techniques will be looked at later in the yoga and breathing sections of this book (see pp. 102 and 120). Yoga, like Chinese medicine, teaches that a balance of masculine and feminine energy makes for balance of the whole. This can be brought about through the physical postures often referred to as "hatha yoga" (*ha* meaning sun and *tha* meaning moon). Yoga also teaches that masculine and feminine energy can be balanced through correct breathing: the right nostril carries the nadi for the sun or masculine energy, while the left carries the nadi for the moon or feminine energy. Both energies then connect and travel down the spine, which is the main nadi.

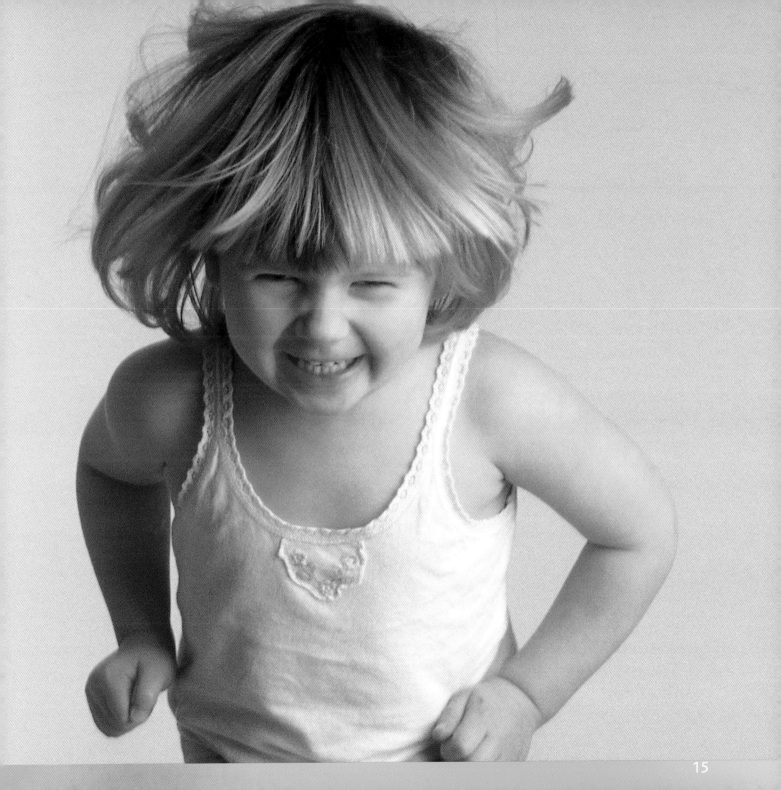

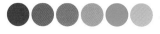

HOW MUCH ENERGY DO YOU HAVE?

When I ask patients at my acupuncture practice, "How much energy do you have?," many of them find it a difficult question to answer. A lot of people will gauge their own energy levels in terms of their friends': Some will measure themselves against a friend who is often lethargic and lacking in motivation, and feel that they have lots of energy in comparison, while others might think that because they cannot keep up with a friend who can seemingly do everything without ever complaining of tiredness, they must therefore have low energy.

This sort of reasoning is not helpful when trying to assess your own energy levels. It is therefore essential, before going any further, to learn never to compare yourself to others in this respect. Everybody's energy needs are different and vary at different times in their lives, which is why it is so important to think about yourself as an individual. (For example, your partner might be able to go out and party every evening only because they work more flexible hours than you do, and can therefore catch up on sleep when you can't.) Concentrate on your own lifestyle and expectations of what you would like it to be, in order to achieve the optimum energy to fulfill it.

To help you determine a fair assessment of what your energy levels might be, answer the following questions as truthfully as possible. They should help give you an awareness of those areas of your life in which you are spending too much energy or not replenishing it, and help you devise some realistic goals to address this.

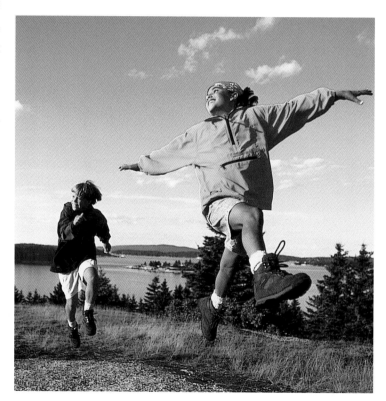

GAUGING ENERGY LEVELS

Here are some examples of how some people say they feel when living with and without optimum energy levels:

With

- wake up in the morning feeling refreshed and ready for the day ahead
- bursting with the joys of life
- motivated
- powerful
- confident and outgoing
- full of a get-up-and-go attitude
- very active, with an extra spring in their stride

Without

- wake up in the morning feeling tired
- simple day-to-day living feels like a huge effort
- everything is a hassle; even getting up from a chair requires an effort
- dips of energy occur throughout the day
- feel aches and pains

By answering the questions below, you will hopefully establish just what it is that you would like to achieve and what might be standing in your way. Now turn the page and take a closer look at some of the factors that could be taking your energy away from you.

What would you like to achieve?

- Do you have enough energy for your current lifestyle?
- If not, what realistic goals would you like to set for your energy levels? (Remember, don't compare yourself to other people.)
- Why do you not have "enough" energy? (Don't worry if you can't pinpoint the answer to this one, but there will be some people who know the cause—for example, poor diet, not enough sleep, etc.—and choose to ignore it.)
- How are you losing your reserve energy (the energy that the body has inherited or made and stored since birth)? Perhaps you are going out late or saying "yes" to a social function even when you are tired?
- What are you doing to prevent yourself from replenishing your reserve energy?

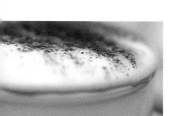

ENERGY ZAPPERS AND FAKE ENERGY

Energy zappers are things that rob us of our energy.

They include:

- stress
- feeling low
- depression
- anxiety
- blood deficiency (mild) to anemia (severe)
- vitamin deficiency/poor diet
- sedentary lifestyle/no exercise
- dehydration, low sugar levels
- excessive work
- eating meals on the run
- being overweight
- lack of fresh air
- inadequate sleep
- emotional strain, worry
- negative thoughts (your own or others')
- stimulants (coffee, tea, sugary food such as candy, carbonated drinks, chocolate, alcohol, cigarettes, recreational drugs)

Fake energy is the energy you get from a stimulant: You feel a rush of energy, but it is not real and is, in fact, stolen from your reserve energy. After the initial rush, you feel even more tired than before and need more of the stimulant to feel energetic, thus creating an addiction. Adrenaline, or emotions such as anxiety, can have a similar effect by generating the same "rush" that an "energetic" person naturally feels all the time.

Trying to manipulate our energy levels by drinking coffee and alcohol, smoking, or taking social drugs and sleeping pills can never work in the long term. Because the "rush" these substances can give you is activated by a stimulant, the energy generated is not real and will leave you feeling exhausted because you will have used up your energy reserve without realizing it. Comfort foods (cookies, chocolate, etc.) and sugary drinks have the same effect: they create a temporary adrenaline increase similar to that used in the body's response to stress.

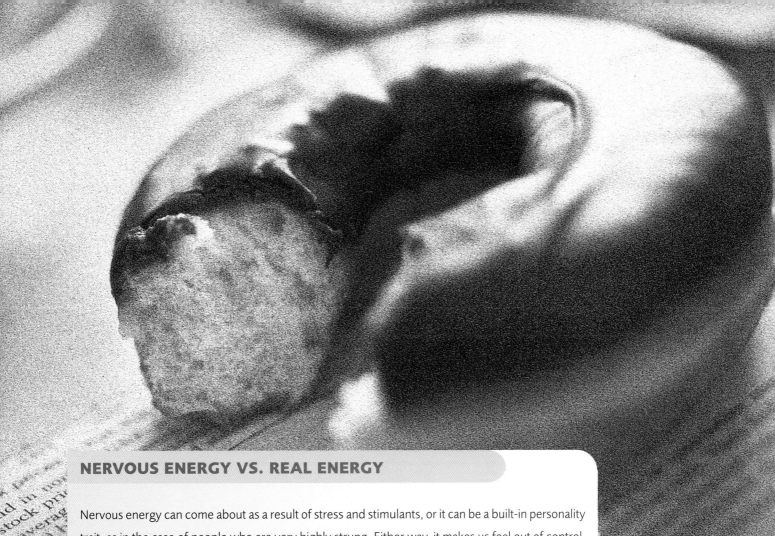

NERVOUS ENERGY VS. REAL ENERGY

Nervous energy can come about as a result of stress and stimulants, or it can be a built-in personality trait, as in the case of people who are very highly strung. Either way, it makes us feel out of control, as if we are on a roller-coaster ride. It makes us feel stressed and under strain, irritable, argumentative, tense, and on edge. Real energy, on the other hand, allows us to lead our lives in the way we want to. Life runs more smoothly with meaning and purpose and we radiate good health and move with ease, with each day feeling like a new adventure or experience. And at those times when everything doesn't feel quite right, real energy gives us the patience to work through whatever it is that is bothering us.

LISTEN TO YOUR BODY QUESTIONNAIRE

1. Do you wake up feeling tired?   YES ◯ NO ◯

2. Are you always saying "I am so tired and I don't know why"?   YES ◯ NO ◯

3. Do you sigh a lot?   YES ◯ NO ◯

4. Do you find life a big effort?   YES ◯ NO ◯

5. Is it an effort just to go to another room or floor in your home just to get something?   YES ◯ NO ◯

6. Do you look at other people and wonder how they have the energy to do so much with their lives?   YES ◯ NO ◯

7. Is just getting up off the chair a big effort?   YES ◯ NO ◯

8. Do you have dips of energy throughout the day where you find yourself reaching for tea/coffee/chocolate for help?

   YES ◯ NO ◯

9. Do people always say that you look tired?   YES ◯ NO ◯

10. Are you stopping yourself from living the life you would like to live because you always/often feel tired?   YES ◯ NO ◯

11. Do you feel tired behind the eyes?   YES ◯ NO ◯

12. Do your shoulders feel too heavy?   YES ◯ NO ◯

13. Do you find it difficult to concentrate?   YES ◯ NO ◯

14. Do your thoughts often lack clarity?   YES ◯ NO ◯

LISTEN TO YOUR BODY Finding an endless source of energy need not be that difficult, and listening to your body is a key step in achieving this. So if you are always saying, "I'm so tired," listen—your body is telling you to take action. If you are not exhausted all the time but sometimes feel tired, you may be running below your optimum energy and in need of a boost.

The questionnaire opposite will help you assess how much energy you have (or lack), and to determine which energy plan would be most suitable for you. If you answer mainly "Yes," then your energy is very low, and one of the longer energy plans would be best for you.

If you answer some questions "Yes" (less than half), one of the shorter plans would be helpful. More specifically, when you know you have a particularly taxing week ahead, you might use the seven-day plan to prepare yourself for it.

Once you increase your energy levels, all other aspects of your life will improve: physically—you will look and feel better and fitter; mentally—you will feel more alert and able to concentrate; emotionally—you will be more relaxed and happy. You will also notice that your work will improve, as you will be less stressed and able to focus better. **Finding energy** So how do you find energy for all the things you want to do in life, and not just what you have to do? Let's start by looking at what gives us energy and what takes it away.

GIVES US ENERGY

Living healthily

Keeping fit

Relaxation

Drinking water

Good posture

Healthy, balanced diet

Good sleep

Good-quality air

Positive emotions

TAKES ENERGY AWAY

Illness

Being unfit

Tension/stress

Dehydration

Poor posture

A poor diet

Lack of sleep

Poor-quality air

Negative attitude

Poor health

Depleted energy can sometimes be the result of a long-term illness, but often we may not even be aware of having the illness in question, having grown accustomed to weariness and fatigue without ever looking into the cause.

The following are just a few of the main illnesses that can cause you to have low energy. I have included stress in this list because being under tremendous amounts of stress on a regular basis can eventually cause you to be run-down and even ill. If you do think you might be suffering from one of the illnesses below, it is important to seek professional medical advice.

ALLERGIES Today, allergies seem to be more and more common because we put our bodies under much more stress than we used to. Antibiotics, food additives, pesticides, stimulants, poor nutrition, alcohol, and drugs all put a big strain on our immune systems, and this has a direct impact on our energy levels.

The immune system responds to an allergen (any substance that causes an allergic reaction) by not recognizing it and treating it like an enemy—releasing histamine to attack it. Allergic reactions take many forms, with typical examples being:

- skin rash
- breathing problems such as wheezing
- streaming eyes, itchy throat, and a runny nose
- tiredness/fatigue
- bowel problems such as irritable bowel syndrome (IBS), colitis, and Crohn's disease
- joint problems such as arthritis.

Tiredness comes as a result of your immune system's constant fight against the allergen or allergens in question, and if the battle continues over a long period of time, you will gradually feel more and more exhausted.

If you can pinpoint the cause of your allergy and avoid coming in contact with it, you will find that your energy levels will increase. This may not always be easy, because we often crave the foods we are allergic to. Eating them causes an adrenaline rush as the body fights the reaction. Afterward, you will feel unwell and tired again.

Tiredness can be the body's signal that it is run-down, and can eventually lead to poor health.

Use of an electrodiagnosis machine (available at many holistic health clinics), kinesiology, or a blood, urine, stool, or hair test can help you establish what you are allergic to. Homeopathy can also help desensitize you from the allergen.

BLOOD DEFICIENCY/ANEMIA

Anemia, or blood deficiency as it is known in Chinese medicine, is the medical term for a deficiency of red blood cells, or hemoglobin. Hemoglobin carries oxygen around the body and contains iron.

Symptoms of anemia can include the following:
- increasing tiredness until you find you are exhausted all the time and feel very run down
- hair and skin that lack life and luster, dry skin, and nails that split easily
- looking pale, with pale nails and tongue
- pins and needles or numbness in your limbs
- dizziness
- floaters in front of your eyes.

If you think you have blood deficiency/anemia, it is vital to get a blood test to confirm this. Bolstering your diet with vitamins C, B12, folic acid, and iron are recommended, and you should also eat foods containing these supplements. A good naturopath/nutritionist can give you more specific advice on recommended dosage and your overall diet. An herbalist or acupuncturist can also help you "build" the blood. Once your hemoglobin levels pick up, so will your energy.

CANDIDA ALBICANS is a yeastlike

fungus that inhabits the gut, mouth, throat, genital tract, intestines, and esophagus. It lives in all of us normally, but is kept in balance by other friendly bacteria and yeasts in the body. Candida gets out of control only when that balance is disrupted, causing it to multiply and weaken the immune system, which results in an infection called candidiasis. Things that might disrupt the balance include:
- overuse of antibiotics, which, over time, weakens the immune system and destroys the friendly bacteria that usually keep candida under control
- taking oral contraceptives (candida thrives when progesterone is high)
- taking steroids regularly
- an already-weak immune system
- too much stress
- too much sugar, alcohol, dairy products, and fried food
- pregnancy.

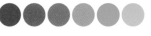

If you have candida in your digestive system, it can also lead to leaky gut syndrome, which occurs when undigested food is allowed to pass into your bloodstream, causing allergies. Leaky gut and candida can cause even more tiredness.

Because candida can affect so many different parts of the body, it can cause a multitude of symptoms, including exhaustion, diarrhea, abdominal pain, bloating, constipation, gas, irritable bowels, persistent heartburn, itchy anus, yeast, bad breath, headaches, mood swings, difficulty concentrating, allergies, food cravings, athlete's foot, muscle and joint pain, sore throat, nagging cough, clogged sinuses, premenstrual syndrome (PMS), and kidney and bladder infections. Because there are so many different symptoms, candida often goes undiagnosed.

Killing off candida involves following a strict diet with no sugar, yeast, or alcohol, and supplements that help restore the balance of friendly bacteria. The actual process of killing it off can make you feel unwell, as toxins are released into the body, but afterward you will feel reenergized. Always seek the help of a health practitioner (such as an acupuncturist, herbalist, nutritionist, homeopath, or naturopath) if you think you have candida.

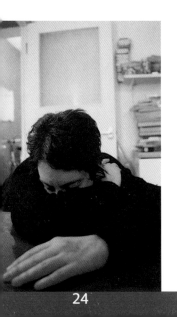

CHRONIC FATIGUE/ME (MYALGIC ENCEPHALITIS) Chronic

fatigue/ME is completely different from just feeling tired all the time. It is a debilitating illness that can occur as a result of a viral illness such as the flu. It can also occur after a shock, exposure to an environmental toxin, or it can even be triggered by a vaccination. Also, if the body is put under more stress than it is able to cope with, the adrenal glands become exhausted. This is also thought to be a common cause of chronic fatigue.

Sufferers of chronic fatigue suffer long-term tiredness and severe exhaustion for six months or more, sometimes even for years. It causes complete mental and physical exhaustion, along with symptoms such as muscle aches and pains, sensitivity to light and noise, confusion, and difficulty in concentrating.

Most chronic fatigue sufferers have to give up work and many of their social activities because of their illness.

If you are, or if you think you might be, suffering from chronic fatigue/ME, you must seek the advice of a physician or other qualified medical practitioner before starting any exercise routines or any of the energy plans in this book.

DEPRESSION Depression is a common cause of tiredness, and one that many people don't like to admit to. People often become depressed when their expectations of life don't match up to reality, or when they are under too much stress. Many people don't realize that they are suffering from depression. It can creep up quite slowly, and it is not until the world feels like a hopeless place that they finally realize that something is wrong.

Symptoms of depression can include:

- having no energy
- feeling anxious all the time
- putting on weight or losing weight
- loss of interest in life/people
- feelings of worthlessness; feeling like a failure
- feeling bored and dissatisfied all the time
- finding it difficult to get to sleep/insomnia
- low self-esteem and no confidence; being self-critical
- difficultly getting out of bed; sleeping all the time
- being very detached from the world

If you are depressed, it is vital to get help from a medical practitioner or counselor. Therapy and counseling can help you deal with the depression, which will, in turn, help with the symptoms, including tiredness.

HORMONE IMBALANCE Hormones can have a major effect on your energy levels. There are many different types of hormones, which are mainly controlled by the pituitary gland in the brain. When one hormone is out of balance, it will usually have a domino effect on all the others, and when an imbalance occurs, symptoms such as tiredness and mood changes can follow.

Disruptions can occur for many reasons such as:

- if you are very stressed
- because of your diet
- through lack of exercise
- if you regularly sleep during the day instead of at night (e.g., shift workers and night owls)
- when there is an illness or physical problem

If your thyroid gland is not producing enough thyroxine, it won't be able to convert food into energy. Symptoms of this condition (known as "underactive thyroid") are tiredness, weight gain, sensitivity to cold, and aches and pains.

If you think you have a hormonal imbalance, you need to have a blood test to confirm it and then see a health practitioner such as a nutritionist, herbalist, or naturopath. Adhering to a regular exercise program can also be helpful.

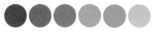

LOW BLOOD SUGAR Sometimes tiredness can occur as a result of low blood sugar, known in the medical profession as hypoglycemia.

Energy comes from food, which the body converts into glucose. We need glucose not only for energy, but also so that the brain and nervous system can function properly. When you eat, this glucose makes your blood sugar level rise temporarily, after which it should then go back to normal. However, if you eat lots of sugary foods or fast-releasing carbohydrates such as white bread, cakes, or cookies, your blood-sugar level rises too high too quickly. The pancreas then releases insulin to bring your sugar level down again, but it can then sometimes drop below its normal level, which can cause:

- tiredness and shakiness
- irritability and mood swings
- nausea and dizziness
- difficulty in concentrating
- regular headaches
- sugar cravings

These symptoms occur mainly between meals or if you skip a meal. This is when most people reach for a sugary snack, but this is the worst thing you can do because your blood-sugar level will plummet afterwards, and you will feel exhausted.

It is important to break the cycle of high and low blood sugar levels. To help you do this:

- make sure you eat every three to four hours
- snack on things such as nuts and seeds
- avoid sugar, sugary drinks, caffeine, and alcohol
- don't eat white flour or white rice
- never miss meals
- always eat breakfast, preferably with some protein in it
- exercise regularly, which helps improve your body's control of blood-sugar levels

You should also seek the advice of a fully qualified health practitioner such as a naturopath, nutritionist, or herbalist.

STRESS Stress is the most common cause of tiredness, and more often than not, most of us don't even realize that we are under stress.

When you are stressed, your body produces adrenaline, making your heart beat faster, pumping blood around the body. Adrenaline makes you feel as though you have lots of energy, but this is fake energy (see p. 18), and is known as the "fight-or-flight" response. This response is mainly unconscious and should only be called upon in emergency or threatening situations. In the past, it enabled people to respond to danger by running away from wild animals or fighting predators. However, running away and aggression are not appropriate responses to modern-day stresses (such as being stuck in a traffic jam, or trying to meet deadlines) and the physical effects that they generate—increased heart rate, blood pressure, and breathing—leave you exhausted afterward.

Regularly stimulating the fight-or-flight response will cause your body to function less efficiently. Constant pressure means that the nervous system cannot calm down enough to reestablish the body's status quo. The body then finds it difficult to relax at all, and after a while you become "stressed out."

People who are under stress all the time tend to do everything quickly, whether it's eating, talking, walking, or other day-to-day activities. In this way, the body is repeatedly depleted of its energy reserves. Once the adrenal glands become stressed, the adrenaline cannot cope with demands that stress is putting on the body's energy levels and is unable to maintain blood-sugar levels. The immune system may then suffer, and illnesses such as high blood pressure, digestive disorders,

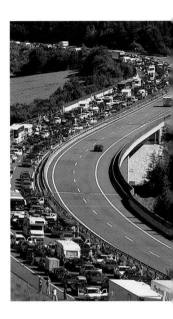

depression, anxiety and irritability can occur, as well as mood swings, headaches, and sleep problems.

This is when most people reach for stimulants to help cover up the tiredness. Coffee, cigarettes, alcohol, sugary foods, and drugs may all feel like they are helping, but in fact they are putting further pressure on the adrenal glands.

Because you become used to functioning at this pace, you may not even realize just how stressed you really are. In order to assess if you are stressed, ask yourself questions like: Am I doing too much?; Do I need more space?; Do I need more time for rest and relaxation?; Do I feel under pressure/anxious/irritable?; Do I find it difficult to relax/sleep? If you answer "yes" to all or most of these questions, you need to take positive steps to relieve yourself of some stress.

Following the simple relaxation and posture, breathing, and exercise routines later in the book can help you unwind and give you the tools to help your body deal with stress. Regular massage, acupuncture, meditation, and healing can also be beneficial. A qualified health practitioner can highlight those areas in your life that you have learned to consider "normal," but which are, in fact, major stress factors.

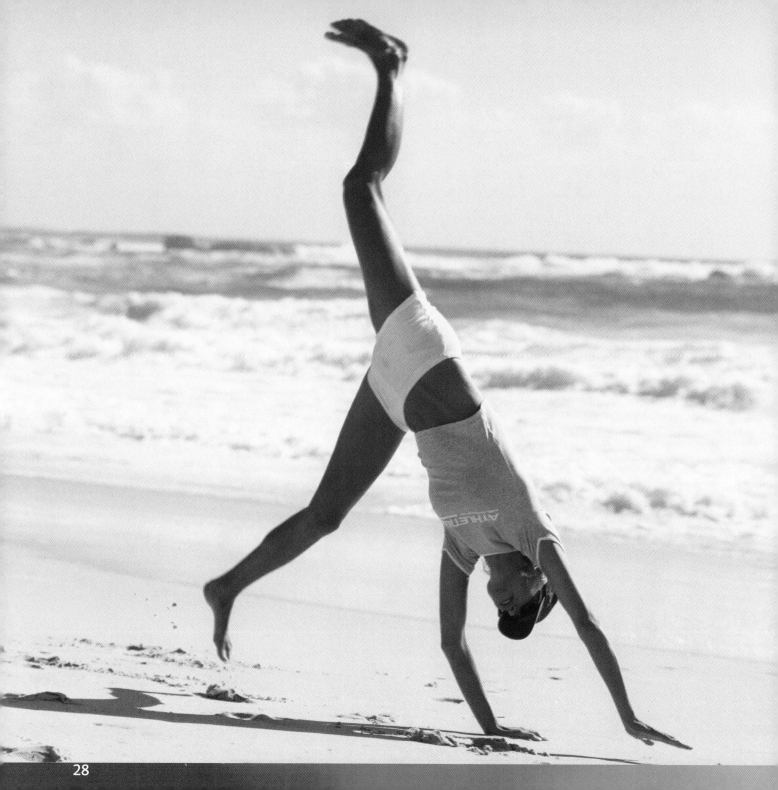

CHAPTER 2
Increase your energy

So far we have looked at why we feel tired and how tired we really are, but we haven't yet looked at ways to treat and beat this constant fatigue.

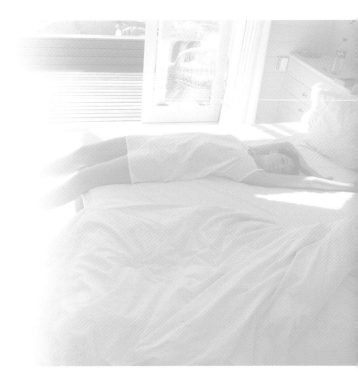

The following therapies can either be practiced at home or with the help of a qualified practitioner (see p. 216 for a list of relevant councils, or ask your physician for a referral). They can help treat fatigue by treating the underlying physical, emotional, and spiritual causes.

Before going to any therapist, always make sure he or she is fully qualified and licensed and has the necessary insurance. It is also very important that you like the therapist you choose and that you feel comfortable talking to him or her about personal matters.

Acupunture

Acupuncture (literally, "needle-piercing") is an ancient form of medicine over two thousand years old, and it is still the most common medical treatment used in China today.

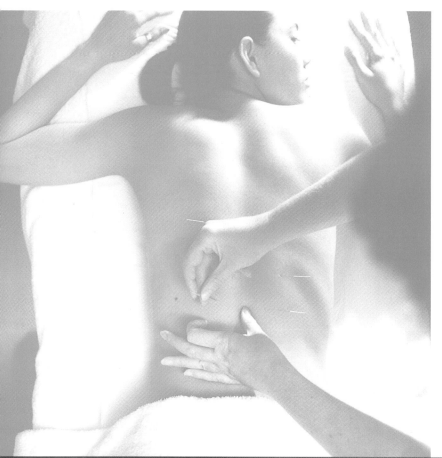

Acupuncture is based on the insertion of fine needles into specific points along the channels of the body. Its exact origins are unknown, but one theory is that when ancient neighboring tribes were warring, men who were wounded in battle found that injuries to specific locations on the body seemed to help relieve the symptoms of various illnesses that they suffered from.

Acupuncture is used to treat disease, for pain relief, and for anesthesia during surgery. Yin and yang, which form the basis of Chinese medicine, are essentially about balance and harmony. Yin represents things like cold, rest, and the feminine, while yang is things like active, light, hot, and masculine. The two are opposites that make up a whole, and one cannot be without the other. They exist in varying degrees in everything; when they are in harmony, we feel good, but if one dominates, it creates an imbalance and we feel unwell. There are twelve main channels in the body, each of which relates to a particular organ. They are divided into six pairs, so there are yin meridians that flow up the inside of the legs and body and down the inside of the arms as they gather energy up from the earth, and yang meridians that run opposite, up the outside of the arms to the shoulders, head, and body, and down the outside of the legs as they gather energy down from the sky.

Through these channels flows qi (pronounced "chee"), which is the body's energy/life force. There are three types or sources of qi:

○ Congenital qi: This is given to us by both parents at conception and is the measure of our overall vitality. It is stored in the kidneys and can be depleted by lack of sleep, stress, and too many stimulants. Dark rings around the eyes are often a sign of depleted congenital qi.

○ Protective qi: As its name suggests, this qi helps protect the body by surrounding it and helping to maintain its natural thermostat so that we don't suffer excessive cold or heat. It also strengthens the immune system. If protective qi is weak, resistance is lowered and the likelihood of illness is increased, which we in the West would recognize as being "overtired" or "run-down."

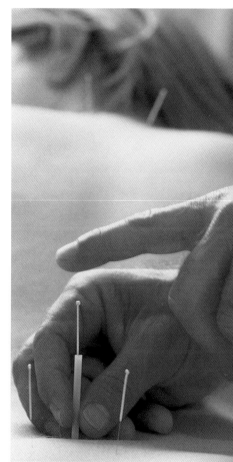

○ Nutritive qi: This is made from the air we breathe and the food we eat. Breathing correctly, eating natural foods, and drinking lots of fresh water help strengthen the nutritive qi. Whereas a nutritionist might say that a particular food is high in vitamins and nutrients, an acupuncturist would say that the same food was rich in qi. In the West we would recognize someone whose nutritive qi was weak if they ate a poor diet and were therefore more susceptible to illness and feeling tired.

Acupuncturists believe that if a person is lacking in energy it can be for many different reasons, including:

○ Blood deficiency (which in its most extreme form can be manifested as anemia; see p. 23)

○ Qi deficiency

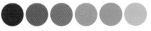

○ Qi stagnation (where the energy has become blocked and therefore stagnant due to illness or stress, etc.)

○ Yang deficiency (where people feel cold all the time, lack energy, etc.)

The specific reason for your fatigue must be established before treatment begins. The acupuncturist will look at your tongue, check your pulse, and ask questions about your medical history, diet, and lifestyle. These may seem irrelevant to you, but will be pertinent in forming a diagnosis. Depending on the diagnosis, the acupuncturist will then choose specific points to work on along the body to help treat the fatigue.

You will be asked to remove certain items of clothing in order to reach the points chosen, and very fine needles will then be inserted into these points and left there for about twenty minutes. People always ask if acupuncture hurts. It doesn't actually hurt, but you can still feel it. You will most likely feel a strange sensation when the needle is inserted, like a dull ache or a bee sting, and this is the qi arriving at the point. When the needles are taken out, you will feel very relaxed and happy, due to the endorphins that are released during acupuncture.

Most acupuncturists will also advise on diet and lifestyle changes as part of the treatment plan and to help you become energized more quickly. While acupuncture is great for increasing your energy, you should not expect to get all your old energy back after one session. You will need a course of treatments (usually between six and ten sessions). It is also great for relieving stress and for treating many illnesses.

If you can't afford to see an acupuncturist, how can you treat yourself? First, you need to think about why you are tired, and to do this you need to look at yourself, and the possible diagnosis, in the way that an acupuncturist might:

○ Blood deficiency: sallow complexion; pale lips; dizziness; poor memory; numbness; blurred vision; insomnia; depression; anxiety; scanty or no periods; dry skin, hair, or nails; tiredness (points SP6, ST36, REN4)

○ Qi deficiency: breathlessness, weak voice; spontaneous sweating; no appetite; loose stools; tiredness (points REN6, ST36)

○ Qi stagnation: a feeling of distension of throat, chest, or abdomen; depression; mood swings; frequent sighing; irritability; tiredness (points LIV3, GB34, SJ6)

○ Yang deficiency: pale/bright white face; cold; listlessness; clear, abundant urine; cold limbs; no thirst; loose stools; desire for hot drinks; sore back; sensation of cold in the back (points REN4/REN6, KID7)

Once you have decided which of the above best matches your symptoms (and there may be more than one), you can follow the points suggested (see diagram for location of acupressure points) and do some acupressure on yourself. Using your thumbs, gently massage the acupressure points using small circular movements; they may feel sensitive, but this is quite normal. When diagnosing, don't worry if you don't have all the symptoms of a particular category as long as you have a few of them.

Note: Pregnant women, or anyone suffering from any serious illness, should always consult a qualified acupuncturist before attempting any acupressure on themselves.

When you visit an acupuncturist, make sure she or he is fully qualified, insured, and uses sterilized or disposable needles only. Nobody should ever use needles on themselves; only allow a fully qualified practitioner to do so. If symptoms persist, see your physician for a thorough checkup.

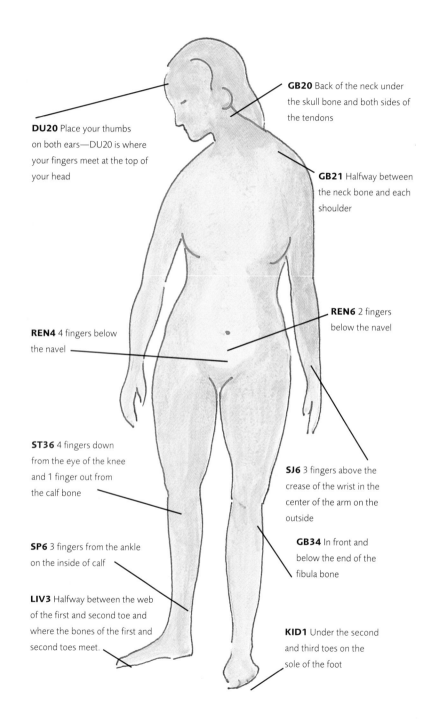

GB20 Back of the neck under the skull bone and both sides of the tendons

DU20 Place your thumbs on both ears—DU20 is where your fingers meet at the top of your head

GB21 Halfway between the neck bone and each shoulder

REN6 2 fingers below the navel

REN4 4 fingers below the navel

ST36 4 fingers down from the eye of the knee and 1 finger out from the calf bone

SJ6 3 fingers above the crease of the wrist in the center of the arm on the outside

GB34 In front and below the end of the fibula bone

SP6 3 fingers from the ankle on the inside of calf

LIV3 Halfway between the web of the first and second toe and where the bones of the first and second toes meet.

KID1 Under the second and third toes on the sole of the foot

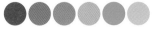

Aromatherapy

Many people think of aromatherapy as a pampering treatment, but it is also very useful for treating medical conditions and great for relieving stress and tiredness. It is a therapeutic treatment that uses essential oils and massage. The beauty of aromatherapy is that it is easy to use at home on your own, though a massage with a qualified aromatherapist is advised at least once a week because regular treatment can help you to stay relaxed, balanced, energized, and in harmony. Hippocrates said, "The way to health is to have an aromatic bath and scented massage every day." But what exactly is aromatherapy, how does it work, and how can you incorporate it into your routine if you can't afford to see a professional?

Aromatherapy uses the essences of plants for healing and the maintenance of vitality, through their unique character, smell, and healing properties. The essences are known as essential oils and are extracted from a wide variety of plants. They are very concentrated—it takes the petals of thirty roses to produce one drop of rose essential oil, and several pounds of lavender to make a small bottle of lavender oil. Essential oils are obtained either by steam distillation or, for the more fragile flowers, by solvent extraction.

Each oil has its own healing property, which can be psychological as well as physical in its effects, and several may be used together to help heal on a mental, physical, and emotional level. They can be used in a bath, massage, compress, or by inhalation, but must never be taken orally.

Essential oils work by absorption through the skin or by inhalation of the aroma. When they are inhaled, they have an immediate effect on the hormonal and autonomic nervous systems that govern our emotions as well as our response to stress. The scents of different essential oils bring about different responses. For example, lavender can soothe and relax, whereas rosemary can revive and energize, and basil can clear the head. The oils can also work by entering the bloodstream, through the lungs when they are inhaled, or through the skin when they are used in massage, made into a compress, or used in a bath. When the blood circulates, the oils are transported around to all the organs. The oil molecules are small enough to be absorbed by the skin, and any that are not used are excreted

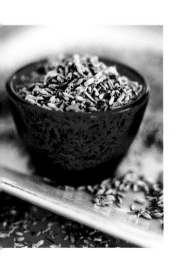

through sweat, urine, and feces. The oils remain in the body for a few hours, but they trigger off a response that can last for days, which is why people say they feel energized, relaxed, and brighter for several days after undergoing an aromatherapy treatment.

The Romans used essential oils for massage and to perfume their homes, while in the seventeenth century, oranges and cloves were used to ward off the Black Death. At the time of the plague in Athens, Hippocrates urged everyone to burn aromatic oils to protect themselves, and centuries later King Charles II did the same in Britain. Doctors who treated plague victims wore protective clothing comprising a leather gown, gloves, and a beaked mask filled with cloves, cinnamon, and other spices. Sponges impregnated with these spices were put under the noses of victims.

In 1937 a chemist named René-Maurice Gattefosse coined the word "aromatherapy," following an incident in which, when working in a perfume laboratory, he badly burned his hand. He promptly plunged it into the nearest bowl of liquid, which happened to be lavender essential oil, and when his hand healed quickly and with virtually no scarring, he realized that lavender

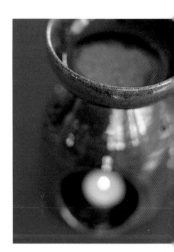

essential oil had better healing and antiseptic properties than any synthetic equivalent. Dr. Valnet, a medical surgeon in World War II, added to Gatefosse's research by using oils when medical supplies were short. Since the war, aromatherapy has grown in many ways, so now the general public is aware of the value of essential oils.

Some oils can invigorate and stimulate while others calm and relax. Modern research has shown that all of them are natural antiseptics, while some are antibiotic, antiviral, anti-inflammatory, antibacterial, expectorant, diuretic, antispasmodic, antineuralgic—all very much more than just a pampering treatment.

Note: Essential oils should be stored in a cool, dark place and in a dark bottle. Most oils will keep for up to two years, but will evaporate if left open to the air. Never take essential oils internally or use them undiluted on the skin.

Always seek the advice of a qualified aromatherapist before using oils on babies and children, pregnant women, or people with any serious medical condition who are under the supervision of their physician.

Massage with oils Massage has been found to be one of the most effective ways of using

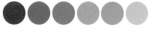

essential oils, since the oils enter the body through contact with every area of the body. The oils are blended with a base oil such as sweet almond, grapeseed, apricot kernel, sunflower, avocado, or wheat-germ oil (the latter being particularly good for people with dry skin). Always dilute essential oils with a base oil; they are very concentrated in their undiluted form and can cause irritation if applied directly to the skin.

Massage of the hands and feet, which stimulates all the zone points of the body, is a good way to stay in good health and help to balance the body's energy flow. For best results, it is important to leave the oils on the skin for six to eight hours to allow total absorption into the system (see pages 50–57 for how to do massage).

Bathing with oils After massage, bathing is the next most effective way of using the oils. Simply run a warm bath, add five drops of oil, stir the water, and bathe for ten to fifteen minutes. This can be done daily to help you relax and revitalize.

Inhalation of oils Inhalation is best used for congestion, during a cold, for example. Pour four cups of boiling water into a bowl, add ten drops of oil, stir the water, put a towel over your head, close your eyes, and inhale for up to ten minutes.

Repeat several times a day if needed. You can also put a few drops of oil on a facial tissue and inhale at your convenience.

Oil burners are available at most health food outlets. Put five drops of oil in water in the bowl of the burner. As the oil you choose gradually evaporates, it not only makes the room smell nice, but also has beneficial effects on your health. For example, lavender makes for a relaxing atmosphere and helps you sleep better. Burning an oil such as eucalyptus can also help in the prevention of illnesses such as colds and the flu.

If you do not have a burner, try putting a few drops of oil on a cold light bulb. As the bulb gets warmer, the oil will vaporize. Or you can put a few drops in a saucer of water and put it on top of a radiator to vaporize and humidify at the same time. You can also put oils on a handkerchief.

Compresses are a comforting and soothing way of using essential oils, particularly if you have aches, strains, or cramps. Fill a bowl with hot water, add six to eight drops of oil, and soak a piece of gauze in the liquid. Apply it to the appropriate area, cover with towels that have been warmed on a radiator or in the dryer, and leave for about fifteen minutes. The compress may be hot or cold, depending on what it is being used for, though heat helps the oils to be absorbed.

Oils to help increase energy

From the list below, choose the oils that best suit or whose smell most appeals to you:

- exhaustion (physical)—clary sage, lavender, orange
- exhaustion (mental)—basil, rosemary, peppermint
- insomnia—clary sage, lavender, chamomile
- nightmares—frankincense
- tiredness—rosemary
- apathy (emotional/spiritual)—jasmine; (mental/physical)—rosemary
- listlessness—clary sage, sandalwood
- sluggishness—lemon, cypress, rosemary
- stress—cedarwood, clary sage, neroli, lavender, orange, chamomile
- lack of confidence—rose, orange, bergamot, chamomile
- depression with lethargy—lavender, melissa, clary sage, orange
- jet lag (to help regulate sleep patterns)—clary sage, lavender, geranium, rose; (to awaken the body and mind)—bergamot, melissa, orange, peppermint, rosemary.

When you go to see a qualified aromatherapist, make sure they are fully insured and registered with a recognized body or council. The first treatment will usually last from sixty to ninety minutes. The aromatherapist will take a detailed history of any symptoms that you have and your medical history, and choose the oils accordingly, taking into account the smells that you are drawn to. They will then mix a blend designed especially for your treatment/massage, and you will need to remove your clothes and lie on a couch in your underwear, covered by towels, and then the massage will begin. After the massage, you will be left alone to get up in your own time and get dressed. You will feel very good, relaxed, refreshed, and energized. Your aromatherapist might suggest further treatments and/or give you a blend to take home. He or she will probably also be able to offer advice on diet and lifestyle.

Ayurvedic medicine

Ayurveda is a Sanskrit word meaning "the wisdom or science of life."

It is an ancient Indian medicine system that has been practiced for over five thousand years. It embodies science and philosophy, and looks at our physical, mental, emotional, and spiritual aspects for good health. Ayurveda evolved from the Atharva Veda, an ancient Hindu book of knowledge containing wisdom about the universe and the secrets of sickness and health.

Like Chinese medicine, Ayurvedic medicine is a complete health care system, and is more than just medicine; it is a way of living. According to Ayurveda, optimum energy comes when body and mind are in harmony and we are in tune with our soul and the universe. It involves advice on diet, exercise, yoga, detoxification, aromatics, etc., and uses a variety of therapeutic tools such as bathing, massage, herbs, mantras, rituals, and meditation to prevent imbalances in the body and maintain good health and well-being.

Ayurveda teaches that every cell in our body is controlled by energy, or prana, the life force of the universe that flows in all people, all living things, and all objects. Prana also controls our thoughts, emotions, and actions, so conversely, every aspect of our lives affects the quality of our energy and therefore our health.

Ayurveda aims to prevent disease by working with your body rather than trying to change it. It looks at the elements (earth, water, fire, and wind) and their related energies: *vata* (wind/air), *pitta* (fire), and *kapha* (earth/water) and believes that health and vitality come from the balance of these energies (see below). These elements determine our constitution, illnesses we might suffer from, our temperament, the type of foods we should eat, and so on. However, in most of us, one element tends to get out of balance more easily than the others due to weather, poor diet, or emotional upsets such as stress. When this happens, it can lead to tiredness, emotional imbalance, and poor health.

What do the elements stand for?

○ Vata: thin build; cold, dry skin; very active and restless/curious; creative.

Unbalanced vata can result in anxiety and nervousness.

○ Pitta: moderate build; fair, warm, soft skin; intelligent; maybe aggressive; clear-sighted; courageous.

Unbalanced pitta can cause frustration, anger, and impatience.

○ Kapha: solid build; prone to weight gain; cool and moist skin; calm with a receptive mind; loving and stable.

Unbalanced kapha can cause laziness, lack of motivation, and depression.

If you are tired due to stress, it is most likely to be your vata or pitta that is out of balance, whereas if you are lethargic and lazy, it is more likely to be your kapha. You can buy specially made teas to balance your energies from most health food stores.

Breathing in Ayurveda According to Ayurveda, without inner bliss (*ojas*) we cannot find vitality. Ojas fills our cells with energy, or, as Deepak Chopra, a health writer and doctor of Ayurvedic medicine says, it "enables the cells to 'feel happy,' to experience the cellular equivalent of bliss." To this end, correct breathing is very important. When we are stressed, upset, or angry, we can often forget to breathe. Deep breathing helps us deal with stress and emotional upset, and also helps to oxygenate the body. Ayurveda teaches that when our circulatory channels become blocked by emotions or undigested food, it causes stagnation, which creates toxins, making us feel tired, lethargic, and lifeless.

Diet in Ayurveda In Ayurvedic medicine, what you eat is also very important, and ojas is only taken from food once it is properly digested. Ancient sages observed how their bodies, minds, and spirits reacted to different foods. They even observed the vibrational energy of a food and noticed how its energy changed from when it was growing, to once it had been picked, and finally when it was cooked. Food is classified in three ways in Ayurvedic medicine:

1. *Sattvic*: foods that promote life, health, satisfaction, and happiness. They help us to be content and calm, and they balance our energies. The sattvic diet includes foods that are usually light, sweet in nature, medium in portion size, and easily digestible. They are calming, soothing, and comforting. They are also fresh, organic, and grown locally. Examples of sattvic foods are: milk (which should be boiled before drinking so it does not encourage the formation of mucus; turmeric and ginger may also be added before boiling),

ghee (clarified butter), fruits (and their juices), sesame seeds, rice, honey, wheat, mung beans, coconut, dates, spring water.

A strict sattvic diet is usually only followed by people who spend most of their time meditating or doing yoga and not participating in the stresses of the Western world. However, if you are lacking in energy because your lifestyle is highly stressed, you can easily help by eating more sattvic foods and by practicing some yoga, meditation, and other relaxation techniques.

2. *Rajasic*: these are very powerful foods; they are pungent, sour, and burning (hot), and make our energy aggressive and overactive.

3. *Tamasic*: these are considered to be dead foods and are tasteless and stale; for example, leftovers or overprocessed foods. These foods make us feel stagnant, sluggish, and lazy.

To increase your energy, Ayurvedic tradition teaches the following:
- enjoy mealtimes; make them relaxed, calm, and pleasurable
- never eat when you are angry and upset
- set aside a time to eat and always sit down
- concentrate only on eating (i.e., do not read or watch television while eating) and eat slowly

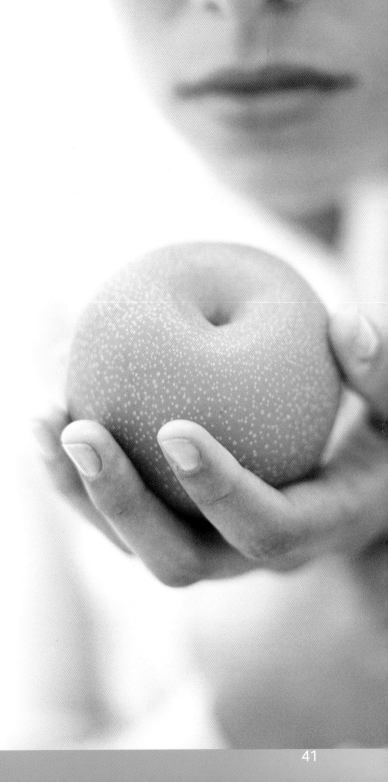

- try to always eat fresh, organic, and locally grown food (as in the sattvic diet)
- try to avoid stale, processed, and convenience or junk food (tamasic foods)
- avoid ice-cold drinks and food
- eat only small amounts of raw food, which is generally harder to digest
- drink warm drinks, preferably not with your food
- eat only if you are hungry
- don't eat so much that you feel you might burst; try to leave a quarter of your stomach empty to aid digestion
- try to have all of the six tastes in every meal (sweet, sour, salty, pungent, bitter, and astringent)
- when you have finished eating, always sit for a while to let your meal digest

If you go to an Ayurvedic health care practitioner, your first session will probably be about an hour long. You will be asked for an in-depth medical history, not only of yourself, but also of your immediate family. You will be asked about your diet, lifestyle, emotions, stress levels, your work, and your likes and dislikes. The practitioner will look at your size, color, shape, eyes, lips, tongue, and nails. He or she will also take your pulse. Treatment will be with massage, steam baths, and herbs, as well as advice on diet and lifestyle. If you can't afford to see an Ayurvedic practitioner, try meditations (p. 76) and yoga exercises (p. 120) for self-treatment.

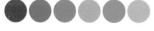

Color therapy

Color can have a massive effect on our mood. The colors with which we choose to surround ourselves, those that we wear, even the colors of the food that we eat, all affect our lives and the extent to which we feel healthy, happy, confident, and full of energy. Certain colors can even influence how relaxed we feel, the quality of our sleep, and whether we have a good sex life. Red, for example, can cause aggression, whereas pink calms.

Research has found that looking at a specific color can actually have a physical effect on different parts of the body. Red, for example, stimulates the glandular system and increases heart rate, blood pressure, and respiration. It has also been found that people with high blood pressure can actually lower their blood pressure just by visualizing the color blue (whereas if they visualize red, their blood pressure soars back up again).

When I was pregnant, I visited a hypnotherapist, and together we worked with colors in a visual way. I was asked to think of pain and observe it from the outside looking in. I was then asked to describe the pain in terms of color, texture, smell, and so on. For me, pain is red and very all-consuming. I was then asked which color would mean not being in pain; for me, it was blue. I then had to observe the pain, turning the red into blue. When I actually went into labor, the pain was strong but manageable. My husband softly whispered in my ear, "Think blue, breathe blue," and it definitely helped me.

What do different colors mean and how can they help us?

○ Red—good for circulation, problems with blood, sexual problems, conditions that are worse with the cold (numbness, etc.). Red is a very strong color, so when you are feeling tired, it can make you feel more energized, and if you feel you are lacking in confidence, wearing red clothes can make you feel and come across as more powerful.

○ Orange—good for depression, hernias, and kidney stones, and can also help milk flow in breast-feeding mothers. Also good for sexual problems. Wearing orange is said to make your sexual energy more vibrant.

○ Yellow—good for digestion, constipation, diabetes, and lymphatic system, liver, and kidney functions. Wearing yellow can help the solar plexus. It is also recommended as a good color with which to decorate the kitchen (being good for digestion).

○ Green—good for nerves, colds, flu, ulcers, and hay fever. Green is the color for the heart (*chakra*), so if you are feeling low or "broken-hearted," it is a good color to wear.

○ Turquoise—good for throat problems and can be anti-inflammatory. When you wear turquoise, you give off a strong healing energy. If you have a sore throat or difficulties communicating, it is a good idea to wear a turquoise scarf or necklace.

○ Blue—good for pain relief, bleeding, burns, colic, respiratory problems, skin problems, and rheumatism. It is a very calming and soothing color to wear. Blue is also great for the bedroom because it helps to induce good sleep.

○ Indigo—good for migraines, ears and eyes, skin, and the nervous system.

○ Violet—good for emotional problems, arthritis, and can also help in childbirth. It is a good color for healing.

○ Magenta—good for the heart and for mental problems.

Color therapists use colored lamps, choosing the right color, filtered in the right amount, to balance a patient, because too much of a certain color can cause imbalances. Each color has a complementary color, and the therapist might use both to get the right balance. You will be given a white robe to wear, and you will sit or lie under the lamp. Light is then shone through colored filters and focused on the area that needs treating.

The therapist will take a full medical history and speak to you about your emotions and personality, best times of the day, and favorite colors. Some ask you to choose the three colors that most appeal to you from cards in order to reveal your mental, emotional, and physical states. They might also make a color diagnostic chart based on the vertebrae relating to mental, emotional, and physical health. The first session may last for up to two hours, and follow-ups are usually about an hour long. At home, you can use the colors in visualizations, or wear and surround yourself with the colors you need.

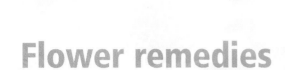

Flower remedies

Flower essences have been used for thousands of years and in many different cultures.

Australian Aborigines used to eat the whole flower to benefit from the essence. Or, if a flower was inedible, they would sit in a group of flowers to absorb the healing vibration of that flower. Egyptians, Malayans, and Africans also used flower essences to treat emotional imbalances. However, most of the knowledge of flower essences was lost until Dr. Edward Bach brought them back into use in the 1930s.

Therapists believe that a flower remedy contains the energy, or imprint, of the plant from which it was made (the Doctrine of Signatures), and that the shape, color, scent, or taste of a plant help to indicate its healing properties. Dr. Bach believed that you did not need to take the whole of the herb, but just the essence of the plant. The essence then goes to work, mainly on an emotional level rather than the physical, thus helping to balance the psyche. From knowledge passed down through generations of his ancestors, Ian White discovered Australian bush flower remedies. I enjoy working with these and have found them to be very powerful.

There are fifty Australian bush flower remedies at present. They are very safe to use, even on babies and animals, and they work as a catalyst for people to start healing themselves. You can self-prescribe; however, if you have a serious illness or find it hard to self-prescribe, it is worth consulting a specialist in flower remedies. The first consultation usually lasts for one hour, during which you will be asked about your medical history, your emotional state, and the ways in which you might react to various situations. At the end of the session the practitioner will recommend the flower essences she or he thinks are best for you and prepare a mix for you. A follow-up treatment will usually be arranged for two to three weeks after the initial visit.

It is fine to take more than one remedy at a time. For Bach flower remedies, just add two drops of each essence to an ounce of fresh spring water, then take four drops four times daily either in a glass of water or directly in your mouth. For Australian bush flower remedies, take seven drops under the tongue morning and night or add the same number to a glass of water and drink throughout the day.

Bush flower remedies

- banksia robur/swamp banksia (for feeling low in energy, disheartened, weary, and frustrated)
- mulla mulla (for rejuvenation)
- old man banksia (for feelings of sluggishness, being low in energy, disheartened, weary, and frustrated)
- macrocarpa (a pick-me-up for fatigue, exhaustion, burnout, and convalescence)
- crowea (for continual worrying, feeling not quite right, and lack of vitality)
- black-eyed Susan (for impatience, being on the go, using up all your energy, and striving all the time)
- kapok bush (for people who give up easily, whose immune system is deficient, and/or who feel constantly exhausted)
- alpine mint bush (for physical and emotional exhaustion)
- dog rose (for treating fears that can be a drain on the immune system and impair the free flow of the vital force)
- jacaranda (for people whose energy is scattered—they start too many things without seeing them through and eventually feel exhausted)

Bach flower remedies

- hornbeam (for lack of energy, listlessness, and uncertainty)
- olive (for exhaustion and burnout)

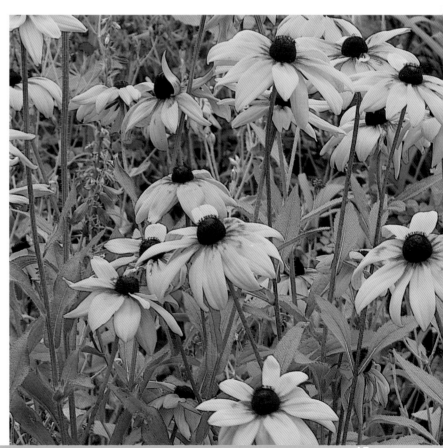

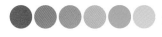

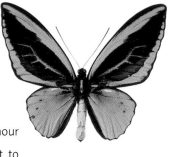

Healing

We all administer healing every day, whether it is in the form of a hug or a gentle rub of someone's back, thinking of someone who has a tough time ahead of them, empathizing with somebody's problems, or rocking a crying baby. Just being held by someone can be really soothing.

You might visit a healer for help with any sort of mental, physical, or spiritual problem—grief or anger can be the cause of low energy just as much as any physical complaint. The main types of healing are hands-on, where the hands either literally touch you or hover above the body. In *reiki*, a Japanese form of healing, certain positions are adopted and various symbols used. In distance healing people can heal by thinking of the person in question when they are not there or through a picture. Some healers believe that they are channeling through a higher energy from gods or religious or spiritual sources, while others believe they are balancing the person's own energy system. Some believe that healers do not actually heal, but open up the body so it can heal itself.

Healers work in so many different ways that it is only possible to say in general terms what might happen if you have a session of healing.

A session with a healer can last from half an hour to two hours. Some healers talk to you first to establish how you need help; others prefer to let their spirit guides lead them to where help is needed. Some like to heal in silence with the lights turned low. Others feel that they can talk to you without disrupting the healing process, and they also believe if you talk, you are helping to release the problems from your physical body. Some will let their hands hover above your body, working in your aura; others will lay their hands on different parts of your body. You might feel their hands are very hot, or you might find the area they touch feels cold or strange. Many healers will report to you what signals they pick up—for example, that an aura feels hot or cold to them. Some might even yawn or burp during the treatment, which shows they are expelling whatever they have drawn out of you. Some healers use clairvoyant skills, as well, and will tell you if they see or hear a spirit or advice from the spirit world. Many people find this reassuring. Others might use crystals.

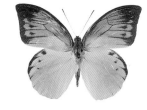

After a treatment you will feel relaxed, spaced out, otherworldly, and reenergized.

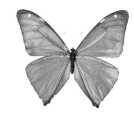

To practice healing on yourself or someone else, you need to understand what it feels like to feel another person's energy. The following exercise should help you to do this.

Feel the energy

To sense the energy, put your hands a couple of inches apart, with palms facing each other. Move your hands slightly like wheels on a train with one hand slightly behind the other in a circular motion. As you do this, you should notice the magnetic pressure between your hands; you can then bounce off the energy by moving your palms slightly toward each other, and then slowly making the distance between them bigger again, making sure you can still feel the energy between them. Your palms may tingle and feel warm. Imagine that energy is coming from the center of your hands. A good device to help you focus is to close your eyes and imagine something opening like a butterfly's wings; as they open, feel the energy coming from your palms. If you prefer, you can ask for spiritual or religious guidance.

You can also practice feeling the energy with someone else. Stand facing each other and hold your palms out in front of you at shoulder height. Don't let your palms touch the other person's.

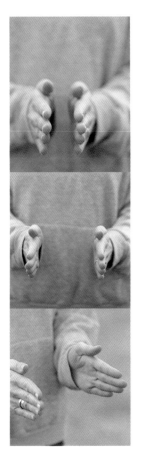

Close your eyes and focus on the energy between your own palms and your partner's. Practice moving slightly farther away and coming in closer. Always shake out your hands or wash them with water when you have finished healing.

If you want to try healing yourself or someone else, or getting someone else to heal you:

1. Close your eyes and either ask for guidance or imagine something opening up (see above).

2. Ask the person you are healing (or tell the person who is healing you) if there is any area that is bothering them, and if so, concentrate on that area. Otherwise, go through the chakras or where your intuition takes you (see page 145 for more about chakras and their locations).

3. If you feel like touching the body, do so. Or, if you feel more comfortable hovering a few inches above the body, that is fine, too. Again, let your intuition guide you.

4. Your hands might feel stiff, uncomfortable, hot, or itchy; if so, just quietly shake them out.

5. Remember at the end of the treatment to either imagine the closing ritual (for example, envisioning the butterfly's wings) or to thank the guides for their help. Shake out your hands, or wash them with water.

Homeopathy

Homeopathy is a safe and effective form of treatment that has become increasingly popular in recent years.

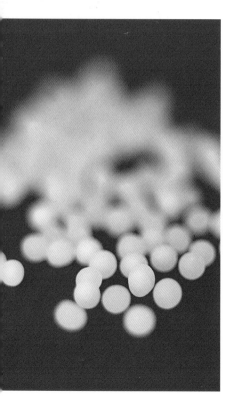

Its name, derived from the Greek words *homoios*, meaning "similar," and *pathos*, meaning "suffering," reflects its basic premise, which is one of similarity. In practice, this means that a substance that can cause a particular reaction in a healthy person can be used in the right dosage to treat similar symptoms or reactions of specific diseases.

The idea is not a new one. It has been around for thousands of years— Socrates wrote of curing a disease with the substance that caused it. It wasn't until the late eighteenth and early nineteenth centuries, however, that it was developed into a formal discipline.

Samuel Hahnemann, the German physician who founded homeopathy, believed that it worked along the same lines as classic immunization: By administering to a patient an artificial illness that has similar characteristics to the condition the doctor is trying to cure. This then stimulates the immune system, the body's natural defense system, to fight the original ailment or illness. Homeopathic remedies produce vibrational reactions rather than physical ones (everything, even illness, medicines, and treatments, vibrates at a certain frequency). They produce a vibrational illness to stimulate the body to heal at a vibrational level.

Many people use homeopathy on themselves, for first aid, on children, or on animals. While it is possible to do this using over-the-counter remedies, it is always best to seek the advice of a qualified homeopath if you are pregnant or if you have a serious medical condition. Always make sure you consult a fully qualified homeopath who is registered with the relevant body or council, and is fully insured.

A homeopath will take a detailed medical history of any illnesses and accidents. She or he will also ask you how you respond to certain situations and

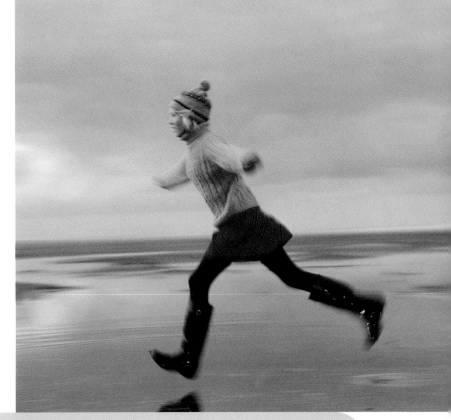

weather conditions, what you are like emotionally, and what foods you like. The remedy or remedies prescribed will be chosen specifically for you based on the information you have given. Remedies consist of a small white pill that is easy to take and may taste slightly sweet or a tincture that is preserved in alcohol. The first treatment lasts an hour and a half, and subsequent treatments are normally about forty-five minutes long. The remedies should be taken half an hour before or after food. Homeopathy can also be used alongside conventional medicine or other forms of treatment.

HOMEOPATHIC REMEDIES RECOMMENDED FOR LACK OF ENERGY

- Kali phos (for nervous exhaustion causing loss of control)
- Sepia (for feelings of being mentally, physically, and emotionally static)
- China (for lack of energy due to loss of fluids, e.g., hemorrhage, diarrhea, excessive perspiration)
- Phosphorus (for feelings of exhaustion following a quick burst of energy, as in hypoglycemia)
- Carbo veg (for total inertia and low vitality, possibly as a result of illness)
- Gelsemium (for mental, physical, and emotional weakness)
- Nux vomica (for lack of energy after having done too much)
- Ipecac (for jet lag)

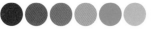

Massage

Massage mobilizes and relaxes aching muscles, but it can also help to reduce stress levels, lower blood pressure, relieve pain, strengthen the immune system, improve circulation, unblock repressed emotions, and increase energy.

Many of us are in a permanent state of stress and tension, which prevents our energy from flowing. A daily massage would go a long way to relieving this, but if you can't afford that—and most of us can't—ask your partner or a friend to assist you. You can even self-massage, using your own hands or a machine.

If you visit a masseur, it is important to make sure it is someone who is qualified and registered with a relevant body or council, and who is fully insured. A practitioner may ask you a few questions about your medical history before leaving the room to allow you to undress to your underwear. You will be given towels or a robe with which to cover yourself. You will then lie on the couch and the massage will begin. Massage is very relaxing, and if you allow yourself, you might even drift off to sleep. Once the massage is finished, the practitioner will leave the room so you can get dressed.

Giving or receiving a massage at home

- Allow between half an hour and an hour for your massage.
- Make the room warm and lie on a firm bed or mattress or on the floor. Your head and knees may be cushioned with a small folded towel or pillow, and your arms should be bent loosely by your sides. Make sure you are warm and covered with towels; the masseur's hands should also be warm.
- Be careful not to massage injured areas, varicose veins, or breasts. Tell the masseur if the massage is painful; they should then lighten the pressure to that area.
- Massage strokes should always work toward the heart.

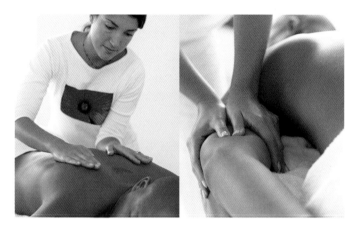

1 Start by stroking up and down the back on each side of the spine, across the shoulders and down the arms, and down the buttocks and legs.

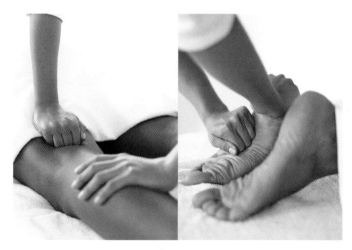

2 Stroke down to the feet and knuckle the soles of the feet; massage the toes between your fingers and thumbs one foot at a time.

3 Do the same again, this time more firmly, kneading and knuckling areas of tension and knots.

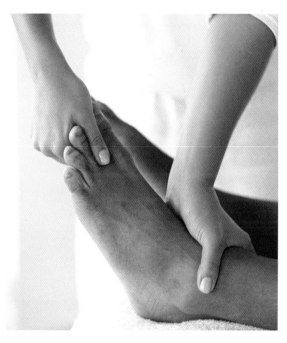

4 Cover the person and let them rest until they are ready.

○ Use oil to help massage; almond oil is good, and you might like to add in a few drops of clary sage or lavender to make it more relaxing.

There are various techniques and strokes. Here are some basic technical strokes you can try (see pictures left to right on this page):

○ Kneading: Gather an area of skin—for example, in between the shoulder and the neck—and knead, pull, squeeze, and stretch the skin and muscles. Make sure you check the pressure—this area can sometimes be tender.

○ Knuckling: With a light fist, knead the area with your knuckles; this is especially good on palms and feet.

○ Stroking: Speed and pressure can vary

There are a number of extra things that can be done separately or as part of a massage:

○ Head and neck massage using circular pressure with the thumbs and index fingers.

○ Face massage: Using your fingertips, perform circular movements with light pressure on the forehead, then go around the eyebrows from the nose out to the temples. Exert a little pressure on the temples and then down through the cheekbones until you reach the nose; then make small, circular movements just in front of the ears

(it might be tender here). Finish by leaving your hands over the eyes for a few minutes.

○ Neck and shoulder massage with pressure and kneading. (Remove any jewelry.) Using the fingers of each hand, stroke each side of the spine in the neck. Start with light strokes and get firmer if you feel you can. Stroke up toward the skull and then back down again.

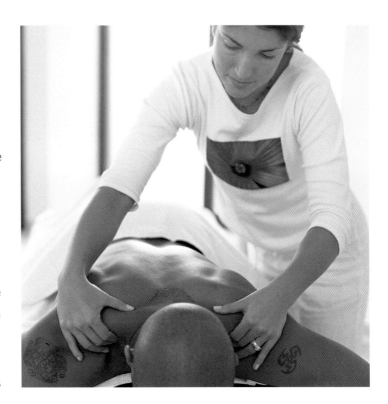

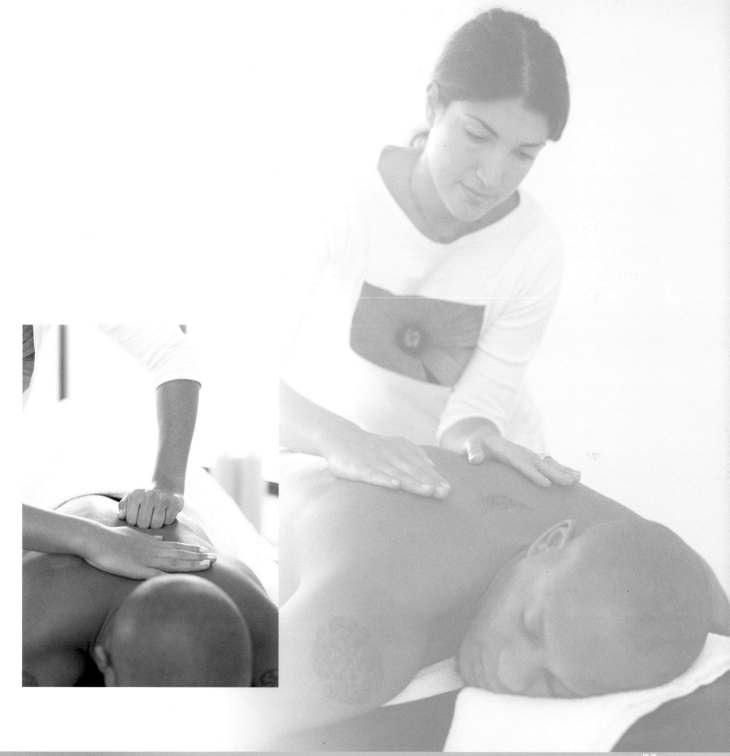

Self-massage is very helpful for reducing muscle tension and stress, and for helping to increase energy. A face massage helps reduce the amount of tension that builds up around the face, eyes, neck, and scalp. Try to do a face massage twice a day for two to three minutes.

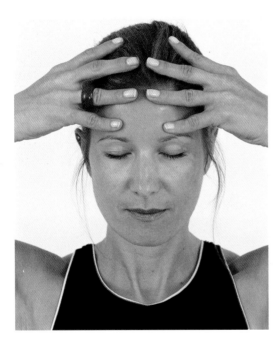

○ Head massage: If you are tense, the skin on the scalp will not move easily. Use small, circular movements with your fingertips from the forehead to the back of the neck. Then work firmly and methodically all over the head, really moving the scalp—as if you were shampooing your hair. This invigorating action helps release tension and stimulates circulation.

○ Face massage: Face and eye massages are good for easing eyestrain and headaches. Be gentle on the face, especially around the eyes, where the pressure should be very light. Use vitamin E oil or almond oil, and if possible, lie relaxed on your back or in a bath or comfortable chair. Close your eyes and start massaging from under the jaw, moving slowly over the jaw and around the mouth, up the cheeks and around the temples, and then across the forehead. Move

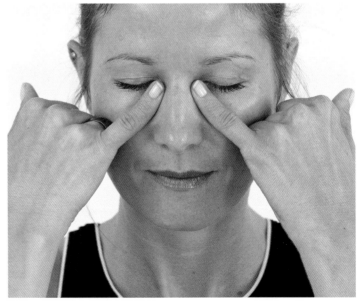

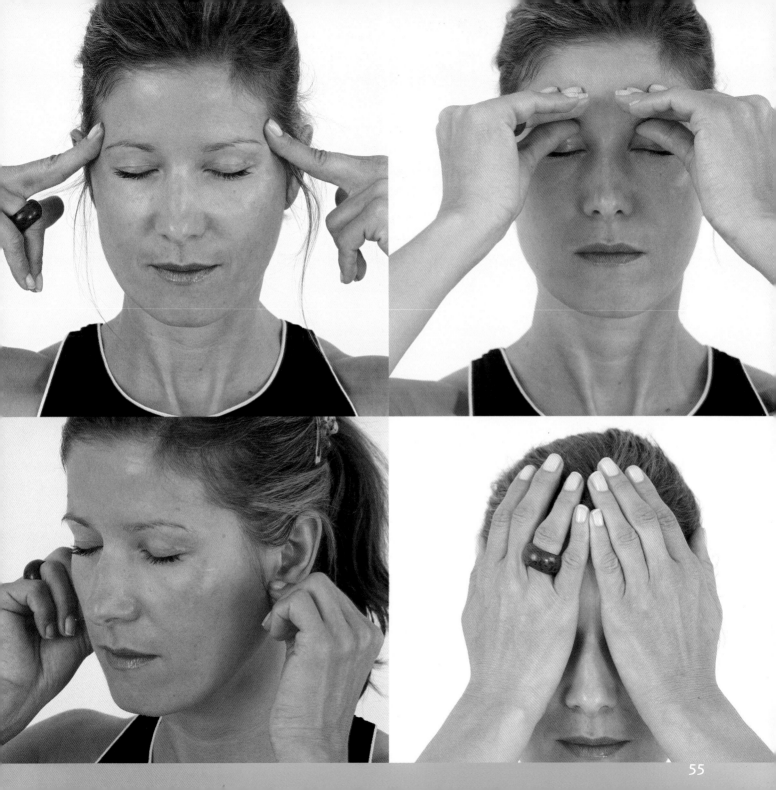

along the forehead from the middle and out to the sides, exerting pressure with your fingertips for a count of three and then moving on until you come down along the eyebrows out to the temples, and down the cheekbones. Use the little finger of both hands and slide up each side of the nose and around the eyebrows. Put your thumbs under your chin, and slide the thumbs along the jaw until you reach the earlobes. Repeat a few times. Pull your earlobes. Then use your index finger to make circular movements in the tender area under the cheekbones and in front of the ear, moving toward the ear. Place both palms over your eyes and relax.

○ Neck massage: Stroke each side of the spine and then work your way up the back of the neck and back down. Use your thumbs to exert pressure on the points where your skull meets your neck (GB20).

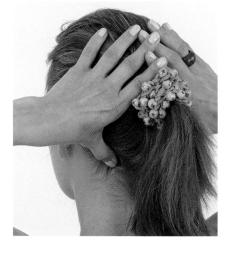

○ Shoulder massage: Using the opposite hand for the opposite shoulder, exert pressure with all the pads of all the fingers. Move from the back of the shoulder to the front. Use constant pressure on the tender points until they are relieved. Repeat for the other side.

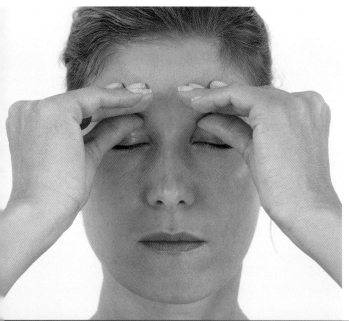

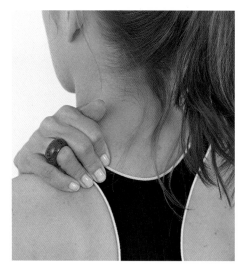

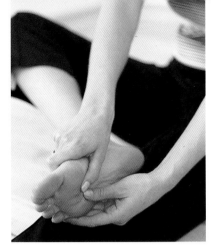

● Foot massage: This can be done at any time, but should be done sitting in a comfortable chair with bare feet. Put your right foot on top of your left knee so you can see the sole of your right foot. Massage the sole using your thumbs from bottom to top, then massage each toe and give each a little pull. Massage between the toes in the web, too, and work around the ankle bones and the heel, and the top of the foot, as well. Repeat for the left foot.

● Abdominal/stomach massage: For abdominal massage, use light strokes, since the abdomen can be quite tender. Make small, circular movements all over with the palm of your hand. NOTE: Do not try any of these techniques if you are pregnant or suffering from a serious medical condition. You should instead consult your physician and a qualified masseur.

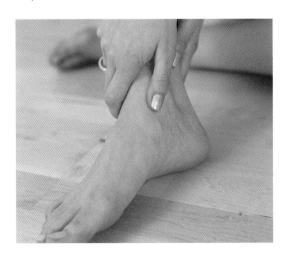

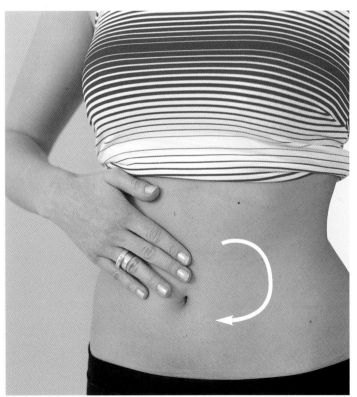

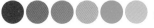

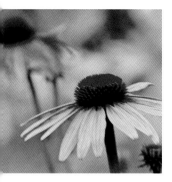

Naturopathy

Naturopathy is a multidisciplinary system of holistic medicine that incorporates diet and nutrition, fasting, hydrotherapy, iridology, herbs, and massage, and is based on the premise that nature heals. Naturopaths believe in using natural resources to get the body to heal itself using its vital curative force to fight illness and disease, eventually returning to a state of harmony known as "homeostasis." The naturopath's aim is to help you achieve and maintain homeostasis.

Naturopaths see illness as natural. They help to identify the cause of an illness, then assist the vital force in eliminating it. A naturopath looks at many factors when someone feels tired all the time, including diet, stress factors, exposure to heavy metals, chemical and electromagnetic pollution, adrenal exhaustion, gut problems such as candida, underlying infections (often viral), imbalances in blood-sugar levels and hormones, depression, anemia, and so on. Naturopaths believe that emotions play a big part in our health and energy. In other words, emotions such as fear, hatred, and resentment can adversely affect the digestive or hormonal systems or blood circulation.

Most of the time, a combination of many factors is responsible for tiredness. However, stress and poor diet are particularly harmful.

Stress depletes the body of nutrients, leaving it unable to function at its optimum level. When we are under constant stress, we give our bodies little time for proper relaxation, rest, and repair. Stress makes the adrenals work overtime producing hormones like adrenaline and noradrenaline to help us cope, but without adequate nutrients and rest, they fail or reach burnout. Eventually, when we require a burst of energy, it is not available.

The balance between the nutrients that we put into our body and the rate at which they are processed has a huge impact on our health and energy. Sugary foods and stimulants are toxic and deplete the nutrients required for adrenal support. Tobacco and smoke exposure should also be eliminated. A session with a naturopath will usually involve taking a detailed medical history and answering questions about your emotional state and lifestyle. They will look at your body type (for example, soft and round, muscular and stocky, or long and lean), which will point toward certain constitutions and illnesses, and may use any of the tools or therapies mentioned earlier.

Reflexology

Reflexology, or "zone therapy" as it used to be called, stems from the Chinese use of acupressure.

The ancient Egyptians also used similar methods, and tomb drawings show feet being held and massaged. There is also evidence of Native American and African tribes using reflexology.

Many people are skeptical as to how reflexology, the application of pressure to points on the feet, or massaging the feet, can be beneficial to their health, but it can be used successfully to treat a variety of illnesses, as well as being both relaxing and energizing.

Each part of the body is reflected in particular areas of the feet, and on this basis, the whole body can be treated through the feet. Reflex points are found on the soles, sides, and top of the feet (see simplified diagram at right), and there are also reflex points on the palms and backs of the hands. The reflex points are organized through a system of ten longitudinal zones that extend through the body, as described by Dr. Fitzgerald in 1913. The zones are divided into five, either side of the central line. Each zone has a corresponding reflex point in the foot,

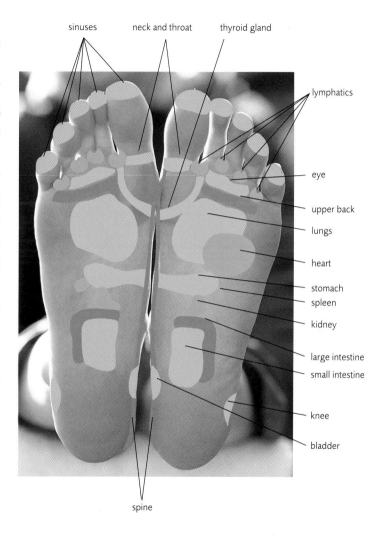

sinuses   neck and throat   thyroid gland

lymphatics

eye

upper back

lungs

heart

stomach

spleen

kidney

large intestine

small intestine

knee

bladder

spine

which the reflexologist manipulates so as to diagnose and treat different parts of the body. In addition to the longitudinal zones, there are also three transverse zones. It is not fully understood how massaging a particular area of the foot has an effect on a corresponding organ, but we do know that it benefits circulation and helps reduce tension.

Reflexologists work with the flow of energy in a similar way to acupuncturists. Because the flow of energy naturally strives for health and balance, it needs help when it becomes blocked to clear, release, and balance the system. By applying pressure to the relevant points on the feet, reflexologists help open energy pathways and release blockages. Reflex points on the hands can also be used, but it is best to work on the feet.

The first session with a reflexologist usually lasts between an hour and an hour and a half. The practitioner will take a detailed medical history and will then ask you to sit or lie at an angle on a couch. You will only need to remove your shoes and socks. First, the reflexologist will examine your feet, looking at texture, color, and temperature; they will also look at the ankles to see whether there is swelling or puffiness. They will then apply talcum powder to the feet to allow ease of movement, and using the tips of their thumbs, apply pressure and perform small, circular movements on the various points, starting from the toes and making their way down the foot to the heel. They will then gently rotate the toes and feet and massage the soles. The treatment ends with a breathing exercise, where pressure is placed on the reflex point for the solar plexus.

A reflexology treatment is very enjoyable and relaxing, and even if your feet are ticklish, you will be able to cope with it because the pressure is hard enough.

You must tell the practitioner if the pressure is too hard, since the points might be tender.

Though reflexology can be done at home, using the map of the reflex points to relieve, for example, a sinus problem, I have chosen to use a basic foot massage in the plans as a tool for increasing energy—it helps one relax and to circulate the blood, and therefore enhance one's energy.

Note: If you are pregnant or suffering from a medical condition, consult a health practitioner before practicing reflexology on yourself.

Shiatsu

Shiatsu is a Japanese word (*shi* meaning "finger", *atsu* meaning "pressure") for a therapy similar to acupressure. It is an Asian massage where fingers are pressed on specific points (known as *tsubo*) of the body to help relieve fatigue, tension, and the symptoms of disease. These points, or tsubo, tend to be areas where the pressure feels uncomfortable because the flow of energy, or *ki*, is blocked. (*Ki* is the Japanese word for "qi" or "energy.") Shiatsu works on the same points as acupuncture, along the meridians through which the body's energy flows. However, shiatsu uses pressure not only from the fingers, but also the palms, knees, forearms, elbows, and feet.

When you have a shiatsu treatment, you can often feel the energy moving along the meridians, which is why it is sometimes called "acupuncture without needles." Like acupuncture, shiatsu can relieve many chronic problems and disabling aches and pains. Like all alternative therapies, it is a good preventative discipline, helping to maintain health, vitality, and stamina. It also strengthens the internal organs and keeps energy from becoming blocked in the channels.

To enjoy a complete-body shiatsu session, you will need to find a qualified practitioner who has had at least three years of training. When you visit a practitioner, wear loose clothing because you will remain fully clothed throughout the treatment, and the practitioner needs to be able to move and manipulate your body easily. The treatment is usually carried out on the floor on a futon mattress. The first treatment usually lasts for an hour and a half and includes a long series of questions about your health, lifestyle, diet, and medical history. Sometimes the pressure points can be sore, and it is best to keep communicating with your practitioner to establish the correct pressure for you. After the treatment you will feel relaxed and refreshed. Like acupuncture, shiatsu is most effective after a full course of treatments. You will also be given dietary and lifestyle advice.

Shiatsu is best from a qualified practitioner, but there are some things that you can do yourself or which you can get a friend or partner to do.

Instinctively, we all practice self-shiatsu when we relieve ourselves from pain using pressure or by rubbing an area that is cold. A mother rubs and caresses her baby when it cries, and animals soothe each other and themselves with their

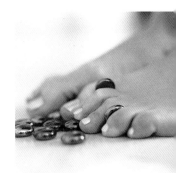

tongues. Shiatsu is simply a more thorough and complex method of this sort of healing (without the tongues, of course!).

When practising shiatsu, apply pressure slowly and evenly; this way, it should not hurt. When you push on a pressure point, use the pads of your thumbs. Press down for a count of five, then slowly release. You do not need to move your finger while pushing down. If you practice on someone else, ask them how much pressure they like. For insomnia the points or tsubo to concentrate on are SP6, KID1, DU20, and, for fatigue, LI10, REN4, ST36 (see p. 33).

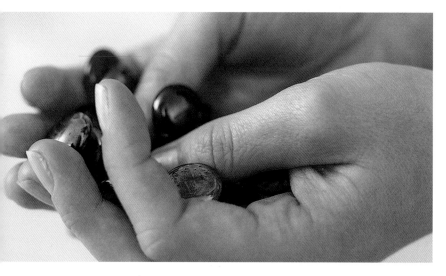

Beating fatigue

1. Lie on your back and put your hands behind your neck.

2. Starting at the top, where the back of your head meets your neck, apply gentle pressure with your fingertips (GB20). Then make your way down in between your neck and the tip of your shoulder and apply pressure (GB21).

3. Breathe deeply.

4. Tighten your whole body and release each part, bit by bit.

No more blues This can help you beat the blues, as well as help to increase your energy. It's also good for stiff joints and bad circulation.

1. Hold some pebbles in your hand, and roll and squeeze them in your palms.

2. Open and close your hands many times and then squeeze the pebbles between your fingers.

3. Put the pebbles on the floor, and with bare feet roll the pebbles under your feet. Squeeze the pebbles if you can and try to pick them up between your toes.

Note: Before working on any pressure points on yourself or anyone else, make sure they are not pregnant or suffering from any illness. If they are, they should consult a qualified shiatsu practitioner.

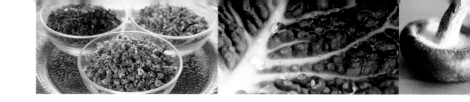

Traditional Chinese Medicine (TCM)

TCM teaches the importance of eating well for achieving optimum energy.

Practitioners can help relieve some illnesses using food alone, or in the case of a more complicated illness, they might use herbs, massage, and acupuncture, too. In Chinese medicine good food is considered to be good medicine.

As in Ayurvedic medicine, the Chinese believe that food contains a vital energy, qi, that is ingested when you eat. Chinese philosophy breaks food down into three main categories:

1. Hot foods (yang): These are warming and stimulating, for example, cooked fruits and vegetables, dried or stewed fruits, carrots, leeks, onions, watercress, lentils, oats, red meat and some cooked fish, pumpkin seeds, sesame seeds, sunflower seeds, chestnuts and walnuts, curries, garlic, ginger, black pepper, cloves, basil, oregano, bay leaf, caraway seeds, ginger, cinnamon, mustard, chocolate, coffee, and alcohol.

2. Cold foods (yin): These are calming and cooling, for example, raw fruits and vegetables, salads, broccoli, cauliflower, zucchini, corn, asparagus, button mushrooms, lettuce, cucumber, celery, eggplant, spinach, squash, cabbage, watermelon, apples, melon, rice, barley, millet, wheat, soya, tofu, mung bean sprouts, alfalfa sprouts, salt, peppermint, nettle and dandelion tea, marjoram, tarragon, turmeric, and seaweed.

3. Damp foods: Create moisture in the body (i.e., if you have a cold, they will make more phlegm), for example, bananas, cheese and other dairy products, and fried foods. Damp foods should not be eaten when it is damp and raining outside.

So, in essence, if you are feeling tired, lethargic, lacking in motivation, slow, sluggish, and depressed, you should eat yang foods to heat and speed you up. However, if you are feeling stressed, uptight, angry, anxious, overheated, and too energized (this might be nervous energy), you should eat more yin foods to calm and cool you down. TCM also recommends that in all cases you avoid leftovers and processed foods.

TCM looks at the thermal nature of people as well as food. Depending on whether you are a cold or hot person, you should eat accordingly. So if you are a hot person, you should eat more cooling foods and vice versa. A qualified TCM practitioner will be able to establish which type of person you are, but here are some general guidelines:

○ Hot person: feels hot all the time; has a red face; is restless, impatient, excitable, hyperactive; walks and talks fast; can have problems sleeping; is always thirsty, especially for cold drinks; fidgets a lot; likes to sleep with the covers thrown off and spread out on the bed; feels hot to the touch; has a loud voice and likes to talk; has dark urine.

○ Cold person: feels cold all the time; is quiet and introverted; walks and talks slowly; is often tired, sleepy, and lethargic; likes to be covered and curled up in bed; wears several layers of clothes; prefers hot drinks and foods; has a quiet/weak voice; does not like talking; is relaxed and easygoing; is vulnerable to the cold; is susceptible to colds; does not like to be active.

○ Damp person: is lethargic/tired; lacks energy; thoughts lack clarity; has heavy, aching limbs; has a lot of phlegm/mucus/pus; has oozing skin conditions; has loose stools; may suffer with conditions that are worse in damp weather, e.g. arthritis; is depressed and listless; has difficulty in making decisions; can feel nauseous.

If you are suffer from a damp condition, it is best to see a qualified TCM practitioner, but just cutting down on damp foods should help relieve the symptoms.

A consultation with a TCM practitioner will be very similar to one with an acupuncturist. Treatment will be with herbs, along with advice on diet and lifestyle.

Note: If you suffer from a serious illness or are pregnant, it is advisable to consult a TCM practitioner rather than trying to treat yourself.

Western Herbalism

Herbalism recognizes the existence of a vital, life-giving force or energy flowing through nature. It also believes that in order to maintain vitality and good health we need to be able to:

○ maintain inner balance (of body fluids, sugar levels, compounds in blood, temperature, and breathing rates) regardless of what is going on around us

○ heal ourselves when we become out of balance

When we experience a physical symptom of an illness, it is simply the vital force of the body trying to reestablish balance. If you feel tired all the time, it is a sign that the body needs to reinstate the vital force that has been depleted. Trying to suppress this with stimulants such as sugary foods and caffeine will further deplete the body's vital force.

It is the job of an herbalist to recognize the body's attempt to heal itself and to support this process with the use of herbs. When you visit an herbalist, he or she will ask you about your medical history, your emotional state, mental attitude, work, relationships, diet, and lifestyle. The herbalist can help relieve symptoms, but will, more importantly, address the underlying cause of the symptoms. The herbalist will formulate an herbal prescription and offer advice on diet and exercise. Herbs can be taken as a tea, tincture (based in alcohol), syrup, inhalation, gargle, poultice, herbal bath, balm, or compress. Make sure the herbalist is fully qualified, insured, and registered with the relevant body or council.

Herbs for energy

○ For stress relief: wild oats, vervain, licorice, skullcap

○ If you are feeling run-down or are recovering from an illness: dandelion, burdock, echinacea, red clover, nettles

○ To boost the immune system and fortify the nerves: garlic, sage

○ For energy and nervous exhaustion: avena sativa (oat extract)

○ For insomnia and nerves: chamomile

○ For low mood: hypericum

○ For vitality: saffron

Note: If you are pregnant or suffer from a medical condition, do not take any of these herbs without consulting a professional medical practitioner.

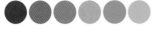

the **energy** plan

Sleep

We all need to sleep, and in fact, tiredness at the end of a fulfilling day is a signal that prepares us for a good night's sleep in order to reenergize ourselves for the next day.

Even when our energy is in plentiful supply, sleep is still very important—without it the body cannot function properly.

An indication of just how important a part sleep plays is the way we feel and function when we are deprived of sleep. We feel irritable, groggy, unable to concentrate, lacking in energy, edgy, stressed, and oversensitive.

How much sleep do we need? Most adults need on average seven to eight hours, but many get by with six or less, while others need more. As long as you are sleeping through the night and waking refreshed and energized, you are getting enough sleep. If, however, you wake up every morning to an alarm clock feeling tired and resentful, it would be best to try to get to sleep earlier, as it is likely that your alarm disturbs you during your deep-sleep stage.

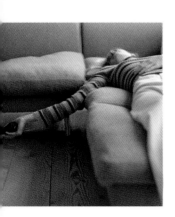

Research has estimated that literally millions of people suffer from chronic fatigue syndrome (CFS). These people find that no matter how much sleep they get, they still feel exhausted, weary, fatigued, and unable to live life to the fullest. If you are a CFS sufferer, you may find that one of the following is the cause of your problem:

1. Illness: Diabetes, underactive thyroid, flu, and many other illnesses can cause fatigue. Check with your doctor to make sure there is no underlying physical problem causing the fatigue.

2. Depression: This can cause fatigue and lethargy regardless of how much sleep you get, and if you are depressed, you probably feel that you want to sleep all the time. Your doctor or health practitioner should be able to help you.

3. Stress: Dissatisfaction with your life and negative emotions can lead to fatigue. Try relaxation exercises, meditation, visualization, and/or seek the help of your health practitioner.

4. Lack of exercise and oxygen: Inadequate oxygen can cause fatigue and sluggishness, as well as a whole host of minor illnesses. Correct breathing and posture, stretches, and yoga will help increase the amount of oxygen going to the brain and around the body. This might just be all you need to help you recover from your fatigue.

5. Holding on to emotions: Regular body massages can help to increase your energy and keep you from feeling tired all the time by releasing stored emotions such as anger and resentment. Some people actually cry during a massage as they experience this release, and afterward they report having lots more energy as a result. Massage also helps with circulation, making the blood and oxygen move around the body more efficiently. This makes you feel and look refreshed, rejuvenated, and reenergized (see p. 54 for some simple self-massage techniques).

6. Lack of fresh air: If you live or work in a centrally heated environment and spend a lot of time in cars, it is important that you spend more time outdoors. Pure fresh air contains negative ions that energize you, whereas indoor and polluted atmospheres contain more positive ions, which make you feel tired. Try to find places full of trees and plants and little traffic to walk in, and keep lots of plants at work. If you ride a bicycle in cities, wear a good antipollutant mask. Keep your home and work cool and fresh. An ionizer or a salt crystal at work or home will help clean the air and take away the positive ions.

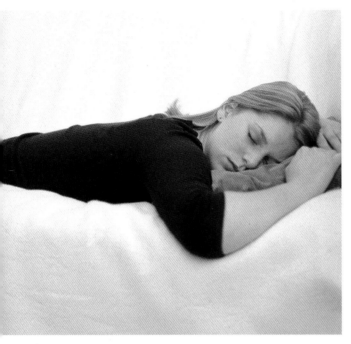

7. Poor diet: Make sure you are eating well, otherwise, you will be lacking in essential vitamins and minerals, which will eventually lead to fatigue and poor health.

Body clocks The body has its own natural rhythm, monthly cycle (men, too), and a heartbeat rhythm. Added to these are the earth's rhythm and the cycles of the seasons, moon, and day and night. The cycle of day following night really affects us since we secrete hormones depending on whether it is dark or light outside. But features of modern living such as late-night parties, birth-control pills, and flying across time zones have made us lose touch with some of these rhythms.

Living life in tune with your body clock allows you to conserve and create more energy. The twenty-four hour circadian cycle dominates our body clock, i.e., sleeping when it is dark and waking when it is light. These and all the other body clock rhythms are controlled by suprachiasmatic nuclei in the hypothalamus area of the brain. When we sleep, these nuclei lower our heart rate, lung function, urine production, temperature, and blood pressure by balancing the body's hormones and chemicals. When we wake up, the same nuclei stimulate everything again, ready for the daytime rhythms to begin (the heart rate increases, the lungs function faster, more urine is produced, our temperature and blood pressure rises). There are also many minicycles during the day, which is why you might notice your energy fluctuating at certain times.

In order to function with optimum energy, it is important to recognize these cycles. Don't try to fight your body at times when you have less energy, and do more energetic things at a point in the day when you have lots of energy.

A typical body clock might function as follows:

○ 12–4 A.M. This is the time for deep, restful sleep. The body is repairing and refreshing itself for the day ahead, so this sleep is very important.

○ 4–6 A.M. The body's blood pressure and temperature are low, making it difficult to work.

○ 6–8 A.M. The brain starts to become more active again as REM sleep occurs, so it is fine to get up at this time if it feels right. Melatonin, a hormone that helps promote sleep, is starting to dip, while cortisol, a hormone that wakes us up, is being released at this time.

○ 8 A.M.–2 P.M. Adrenaline is rising, so this is when the brain is most alert. This is a good time to get a lot of work done, especially mental work.

○ 2–5 P.M. Energy levels can start to dip during these hours, so it is a good time to eat lunch and to perform tasks that require less energy or concentration.

○ 5–6 P.M. The muscles are warm and the heart and circulation are working at their best, so this is a very good time to exercise.

○ 6–8 P.M. The sleep hormone starts to be released around now, so you will begin to feel more relaxed and tired. In the summer this will be slightly later since it gets dark later.

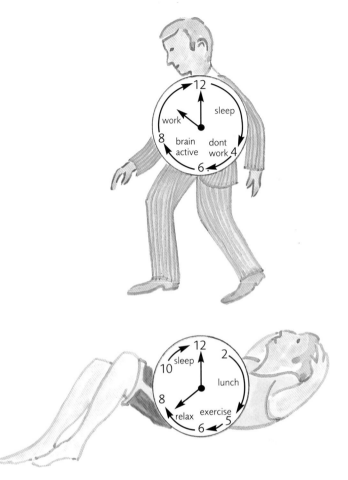

○ 10–12 P.M. This is the best time to go to sleep because melatonin levels are high. This means you will be asleep in time for the deep sleep around midnight—in preparation to wake up refreshed the next day.

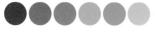
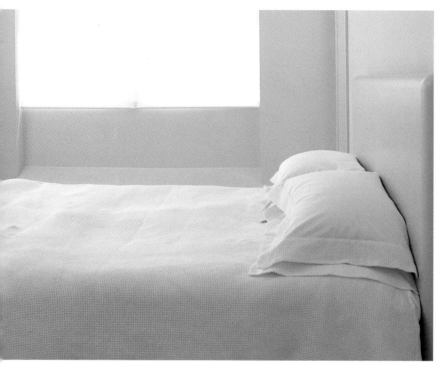

This is a very average body clock, and not everybody does or should work in this way. There are many reasons why one person's body clock may not fit into the typical pattern, such as frequent travel to different time zones, but the important thing is that your body clock suits your lifestyle and works for you. If, however, you feel that you would like to reestablish your body clock to maximize your energy levels, it is possible to reprogram it.

To reprogram your body clock to fit the standard pattern, simply set an alarm to go off at the same time, early every morning until you are waking up before it goes off. You must get out of bed as soon as you wake up. Do this for another week, and your new body clock should be set.

JET LAG–BUSTERS

○ To help regulate sleep patterns when traveling, try essential oils of clary sage, lavender, geranium, or rose.

○ To awaken the body and mind, try bergamot, melissa, orange, peppermint, rosemary, or ginger.

○ The Australian bush flower remedy Travel Essence may be taken before and during travel and on arrival. It really does help.

Getting to sleep Some people find that no matter what time they go to bed, they still have difficulty falling asleep. Here are some suggestions:

- Avoid caffeine after 5 P.M. and, if possible, cut down on the amount you have during the day. Ideally, you should cut it out completely.
- Drink a cup of chamomile tea or valerian tea before going to bed.
- If you can't sleep, get out of bed and do something else; don't toss and turn in bed, because your body needs to recognize that your bed is for sleeping.
- Don't read in bed or watch television, since that will stimulate you.
- Have a hot bath before bed with a few drops of lavender, juniper, and marjoram oils.
- Try some relaxation exercises, either in bed or in the bath.
- Try playing some soothing background music.
- Eat a couple of hours before going to bed so you don't go to bed hungry.
- If you can't sleep because you are worrying over things that need to be done the next day, go into another room and write down all the things you need to do. That way you should feel more relaxed knowing that everything is on a list and won't be forgotten.

And here are a few more tips to help you enjoy more good-quality sleep once you've managed to fall asleep consistently:

- Try going for a walk every day.
- Before going to bed, write a list of things to do the next day.
- Avoid sleeping medications. They do not address the root cause of your problem, and they also suppress REM sleep, which is essential for good health. Try a natural alternative such as valerian, which is nonaddictive and helps promote healthy sleep patterns.
- Make sure your bed is comfortable and that the room has a soothing, relaxing atmosphere.
- Never leave the heating on overnight. It will make you wake up tired and sluggish.
- Avoid big meals before bed. A light meal of calcium-rich foods around two to three hours before you go to bed is recommended. (These foods are known as nature's tranquilizers.)

Sleep and stress When we are under a lot of pressure, we experience stress. This can leave us feeling quite exhausted by the end of the day, and if the stress continues over a period of time, we can really be drained of energy. When we take steps to relieve stress, we give the body time to recharge. Think back to your last vacation and how much energy you had when you got home.

Regular relaxation exercises and activities can help enormously to counteract the effects of stress, but just being aware of when your body is under stress is a vital key to stress-busting. Stress

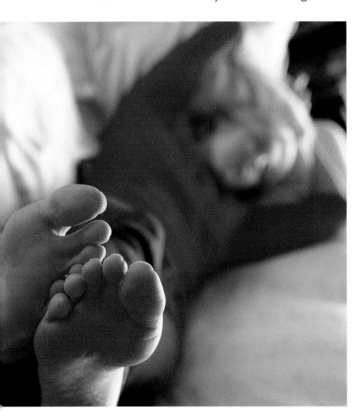

factors need not only be negative things such as bereavement, divorce, or losing a job. Many positive things such as getting married, moving into a new house, or even going on vacation can induce huge amounts of stress. As a result, many people in today's busy world are unaware of just how stressed they really are. Try answering the following stress questionnaire to find out how much stress you are carrying:

1. Do you have difficulty sleeping or trouble staying asleep?

2. Do you feel anxious a lot of the time?

3. Do you often have a stiff neck and shoulders?

4. Do you grind your teeth at night?

5. Is your jaw clenched tight even now?

6. Are you constantly going over things in your mind repeatedly?

7. Do you find it difficult to stop, relax, and clear your mind?

8. Do you find that you need alcohol, cigarettes, or social drugs to help you relax?

9. Do you have problems with your skin or digestion?

10. Are you offended easily and have mood swings for no apparent reason?

11. Do you eat and talk quickly, and want people

to tell you things quickly so you can move on?

12. Does your leg shake under the table when you are working or sitting down at a meal?

13. Do you feel that there is not enough time in the day for everything?

14. Do you long for a vacation, a break from your daily routine, or a change of lifestyle?

If you have answered "yes" to most of these questions, you are carrying a lot of stress.

When you are stressed, the quality of your sleep is diminished. Quality sleep contains adequate REM and deep non-REM sleep. REM sleep is light dream sleep, when the brain sorts through all of your daily activities and thoughts. Deep sleep is when the body repairs itself and growth and sex hormones are released. With sufficient amounts of both types of sleep, you will wake up feeling refreshed and raring to go. It is therefore essential to try to relieve any stress you may have before going to bed.

RELAXING THE TENSION BEFORE BED

Regular relaxation exercises and/or alternative therapies will help you get a good night's sleep. Massage, deep breathing, stretching, and yoga will all help to relax your brain and calm your body, especially if you do them before going to sleep.

Try the following exercise every night when you get into bed. It's great if you are feeling stressed and/or can't sleep:

1. Lie down with the lights off. Close your eyes and innocently observe your breathing (see p. 76).

2. When you are ready to begin, tense each part of your body individually, starting with your toes, then your feet, calves, knees, all the way up to your eyes, nose, cheeks, and top of your head.

3. Starting with your toes, hold the tension and then release, exhale and move on to the next part of your body. Notice the difference between holding the tension and relaxing.

4. When you have done your whole body, front and back, top and bottom, you should (if you're not asleep already!) feel very relaxed.

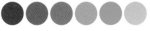

Relaxation techniques

Learning to relax both physically and mentally is a crucial skill.

It is equally important to find the relaxation technique that works for you. If you are an impatient person, for example, you should try a short relaxation technique. When a relaxation method works, you will feel physical benefits: Your heart rate slows down, your blood pressure falls, and your breathing becomes slower and more rhythmic. Your saliva and bile are also stimulated to aid proper digestion, allowing your bodily functions to work properly. You will also feel calmer.

When you feel calm, your mind works at its best. Concentration and memory improve. You see problems in perspective, and you feel lighter, stronger, and more centered. You are able to let go of emotions such as anger and frustration, allowing your body to recharge and create new energy.

Learning to unwind at the beginning, middle, and end of each day gives you a simple tool with which to help your body cope better and to give you more real energy throughout the day.

During a meditation or visualization, your heart rate and breathing slow down, the bronchi of the lungs dilate, blood pressure drops, and the production of stomach acid is reduced. Most importantly, no stress hormones are released into the bloodstream. Relaxation exercises (including visualization and meditation) are not the same as sleeping, because during a meditation and/or visualization, the brain emits alpha waves, showing the brain to be mentally alert but physically relaxed.

Meditation Being in a meditative state is actually very similar to what we might call "daydreaming"; we all switch in and out of simple meditative states throughout the day without even realizing it. I have included the walking meditation on page 77 to show how a "normal" meditative activity can be enhanced simply by increasing awareness, and to take away many peoples' fear of meditation.

When you meditate (as with visualizations or relaxation exercises), you turn your attention inward. Even though you are aware of where you are, it is no longer at the center of your mind. Meditation helps you find inner peace by calming the mind and helping it to focus. It provides a rare opportunity to find a little space in a hectic world—and often a hectic mind.

Meditation requires practice and discipline. When you meditate, you let go of your thoughts just for the time of the meditation, in the knowledge that you can think about them all again when the meditation is over. The mind loves to be active, and it is very easy to get swept along on a daily basis by your thoughts and emotions, but this can be very tiring. The first step of meditation, then, is to become aware of how busy your mind is—and then learn to let it go.

During everyday activities, the brain operates on fast theta waves, but when you meditate, the brain waves change to the slower alpha waves that occur with relaxation. Experienced meditators can even experience delta waves similar to those activated during sleep.

There are many activities that we do on a daily basis that are quite meditative, such as cycling, cleaning, painting, or anything where the mind is used in a disciplined way so it can't wander off into a whole chain of thoughts.

It can take weeks or even months to really see the benefit of meditation, so don't give up too soon. Once you have found the meditation that works well for you, try to stick to it and use the same method every day. The walking meditation below is a good example of a simple activity that has a meditative quality.

Rules for doing any relaxation technique:

1. Find a quiet space in which to relax (this can even be the restroom if you are at work), preferably first thing in the morning, at noon, or when it gets dark. Avoid doing it immediately after a meal.

2. Turn off all phones.

3. Ask your family/colleagues not to disturb you.

4. Make yourself comfortable (for example, sit on a chair with your feet resting on the floor).

5. Try to use the same place at the same time every day so your body gets into a routine.

6. Tell yourself to let go of your worries for just ten to twenty minutes; you can think about them all again when the exercise is finished.

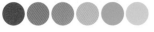

Simple meditations

⦿ Breath meditation:

1. Sit comfortably on a chair or lie down.

2. Close your eyes and slowly focus your attention on your breathing. Don't judge your breathing by thinking it's too fast or too slow; just observe it objectively.

3. Every time your mind wanders, which it most certainly will do, just let the thought go (you can always think about it later) and go back to observing your breathing.

At first you might find it difficult to stop your mind from wandering, especially if you are stressed and/or very busy, but with practice you will find that you might have just one second or minute when your mind is clear, and this will feel like bliss. You can do this meditation anywhere, anytime: on a train or a bus, or in a waiting room.

⦿ Mantra meditation:

1. Pick a word or phrase that you like like, such as "peace," "love," "health," or "energy," and repeat it over and over either in your head or aloud. This word is your mantra. The traditional Hindu mantra is "om," said to be the sound of the whole universe, and it will help you bring about changes in your real self. It is also very balancing

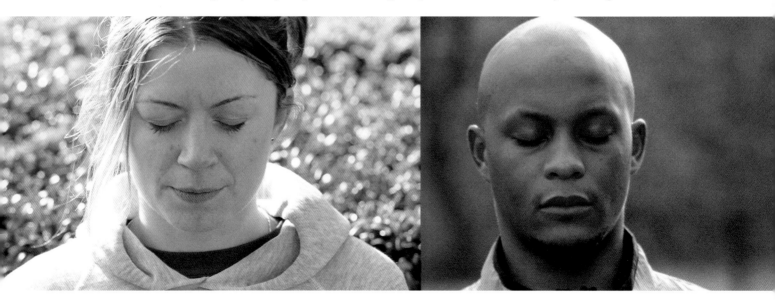

and massages the internal organs, increases blood flow, stimulates the nervous system, and relaxes the respiratory system.

2. Close your eyes and take a few deep breaths when you are ready to start.

3. Concentrate and focus on your chosen word or phrase. Still your mind and turn your attention inward. By doing this you will focus your mind on your inner world and find a state of peace.

This type of meditation is particularly good if you find it difficult to stop the constant internal dialogue, as it helps you focus the mind.

○ Walking meditation

1. As you walk, become aware of your feet.

2. Begin by saying in your head, "left right left right," then just let the rhythm take you into a meditative state. If any problems are bothering you, try to put them aside until after the walk.

Visualizations To visualize means to see something in your mind's eye, which we all do instinctively every day. If someone stops to ask you for directions, you will visualize the route in your mind; if you are thinking about what you did last night, you visualize the evening in your mind. When you listen to the radio or hear someone describing something, or even when you read a

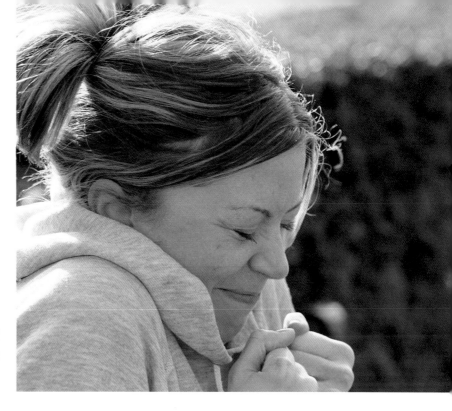

book, you will automatically produce pictures in your mind. In fact, when you see a film based on a book that you have read, you are often disappointed because the characters in the film do not look as you'd visualized them.

So if you feel that you have "no imagination" and worry that you will not be able to visualize, fear not. Everyone can visualize, and everyone does!

A good friend of mine, Pete Cohen, who does NLP (Neuro-Linguistic Programming) and also wrote the foreword to this book, once told me that the key to visualization is not to concentrate too hard with your mind. This really helped me to relax and stopped me from constantly trying to force my mind to think of the image I wanted to see.

Earth's energy Allow yourself at least fifteen to twenty minutes for this visualization:

1. Close your eyes and innocently observe your breathing objectively (see p. 76).

2. Imagine yourself sitting under a big, old tree. Feel your back supported by its trunk as you lean against it. Continue to observe your breathing.

3. With your feet on the ground, feel the earth's energy pull your stress out through your feet. Observe your breathing again.

4. When you are beginning to feel relaxed, allow the energy of the earth and tree to fill your body, starting with your feet and working its way up your body, through your back right up into the top of your head. Your feet will probably tingle, and you may feel like you have butterflies in your stomach as you start to recharge your batteries.

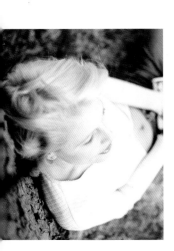

5. When you are ready and feel that your energies have been recharged, slowly come back to the room and open your eyes.

Ten-minute sun meditation This is designed to be a ten-minute exercise, but if you can find twenty minutes, so much the better:

1. Find a chair to sit on, preferably a comfortable one (although even a toilet will do if necessary.) Close your eyes and begin to observe your breathing objectively (see p. 76).

2. Empty your mind. If you find this difficult, when and if a thought comes into your mind, tell yourself to let it go, and you can think about it in ten (or twenty) minutes.

3. Once you have started to relax, revisit a beautiful beach, park, or waterfall in your mind. Allow the energy of nature to recharge you. Remember how good it feels to bask in the sun. Feel the sun warming your face and tickling your body from your head to your toes. Let it calm and reenergize you. Keep observing your breathing. Bask in the sun for as long as you can or want.

4. When you are ready, slowly open your eyes.

When you get used to doing this, you will find that you can even meditate on a busy train or bus. But to begin with, do the sun meditation in the morning when you wake up, at midday, or when you get back from work. If your day is very stressful, take ten minutes out just to recharge.

Relaxation exercises

Relaxation exercises are simply exercises that make you relax the muscles in a particular way, or make you conscious of how you are holding stressed muscles.

Relax anytime, anywhere

1. Take a deep breath in and clench all your muscles.

2. Make a fist with your hands, tighten your jaw, scrunch up your face, lift your shoulders up to your neck as seen in the picture at right, tighten your bottom, curl your toes.

3. Hold all these positions for a few minutes and then breathe out fully and relax every muscle, letting every bit of tension out with your breath.

4. Breathe normally, then repeat a couple of times.

Stressbuster

1. Lift your shoulders up and down a couple of times, then rotate them forward and backward a few times.

2. Close your eyes and concentrate on your breathing.

3. When you are breathing deeply, look up and stretch your arms above your head. Stretch

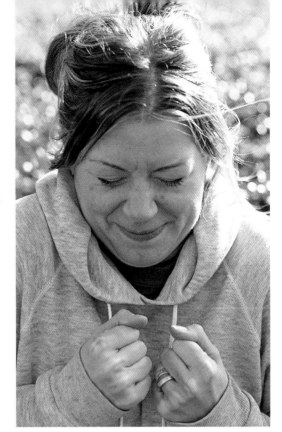

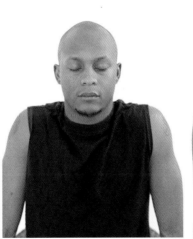

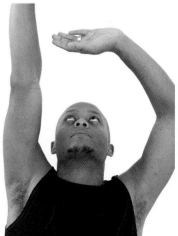

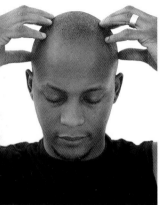

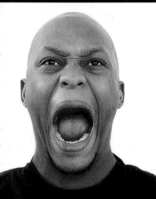

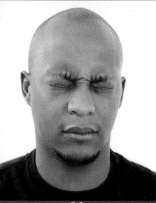

higher with one hand first, then repeat with the other hand.

4. Rub your head and then tap it with your fingertips; tug your hair and then release your hands.

5. Squeeze around your jaw and then tap it to release the tension often held there, especially if you grind your teeth.

6. Clench your jaw and then open wide and say, "Aaaahhhhh."

7. Squeeze your eyes shut and then open them wide.

8. Close your eyes and breathe through your nose while imagining something very peaceful, such as a beach at sunset.

Ease the tension

This exercise can also be done anywhere, anytime.

1. Close your eyes.

2. Place your thumb and index finger on your eyebrow and squeeze it between them, starting at the nose and moving outward.

3. With your thumbs, push down for a count of five and then move along the bone, under your eyebrow, again starting at the nose.

Private release of tension

1. Stand with your feet hip width apart.

2. With your arms at your sides, shake out your hands and then your arms.

3. Roll your shoulders forward six times and then backward six times.

4. Roll your neck from side to middle to side, first one way and then the other.

5. Shake your head as if saying "no" and while letting your face relax completely, allow a strange warbling sound to come from your relaxed mouth and cheeks.

6. Lift up one foot and shake it, then shake out your leg; repeat with the other leg.

7. Put your hands on your hips and move your hips in a circle one way and then the other. Move your pelvis backward and forward.

8. With your feet remaining hip width apart and your knees bent, clasp your hands together.

9. Lift your arms above your head and breathe in. Exhale and shout "ha" while swinging your arms down, as if you were chopping wood, and between your legs.

10. Swing your arms back up again until you are standing upright.

Repeat as many times as you feel is necessary.

Mental attitude

When looking at energy, we are more than just our physical bodies. What happens to us emotionally and psychologically is reflected in physiological changes in our bodies. Taking this into account, it is then obvious that our energy levels will also be affected by mental attitude, the way in which we relate to others, and whether we are enjoying life or finding everything a struggle.

Just as negative emotions can zap your energy, learning to love and feeling positive emotions can boost it. Liking yourself is also very important. A poor, negative self-image can really drain your energy, and by constantly criticizing yourself, you use up energy that could have been applied to other things.

To achieve a positive mental attitude:

○ Try to see a positive outcome to every situation.

○ If something doesn't happen that you wanted—for example, you don't get a job that you were hoping to get—remember the phrase, "It obviously wasn't meant to be; something better will be waiting around the corner."

○ Give yourself compliments and confidence-boosts: "I am a nice person," "I am talented and good at art/self-expression/writing poetry," "I am a good listener," etc. It is even helpful to make a list of these things so you can look at it whenever you feel yourself starting to become negative or self-critical.

○ Every time you catch yourself being negative, turn the situation or sentence around and change it into a positive one.

○ Make choices for your own life; don't just accept what comes to you because you believe you don't deserve any better.

○ Start the day with an activity that you like, for example, reading with a cup of herbal tea.

○ Do something you have never done before and thought you could never do, like skydiving, in-line skating, acting classes, or surfing.

○ Surround yourself with positive people.

○ Repeat positive mantras (see p. 76) to yourself whenever you catch yourself being negative: "I have loads of energy and can do anything that I choose to do in life"; "I know that every day and in every way I am getting better and better"; "Throw it away, throw it away, let it go, let it go"; "If I will it, it is no dream"; "I can do anything."

○ Always remember that you are unique, and only you can do the things you do.

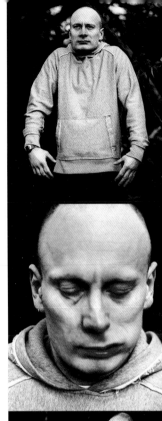
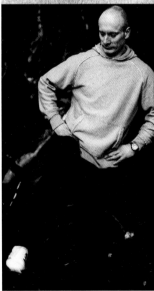

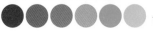

Structured time

Many people take their work home with them, either literally, when they do not have enough hours in the working day to get through it all, or figuratively, simply by worrying about it after hours. When you are working on energy levels, it is very important to set structured times for work so there is always time to unwind.

In order to structure your time, a "to-do" list is a must. Otherwise, before you know it, a firm intention becomes yet another thing you wanted to do, but work and other things got in the way.

We all spend a lot of energy trying to remember things that we have to do and worrying about doing them. Writing a to-do list helps us stop worrying; it allows us to stop carrying around lots of jobs and worries in our head so we can spend that energy either on getting those jobs done or using it elsewhere.

Try to write your lists every morning or every afternoon, whichever works best for you. You may find that you don't need to do it daily and that a weekly list that you can add to on a daily basis works better. Some people like to include sections such as "work," "home," and "personal."

Try to prioritize the various jobs and write in your diary when you plan to do them. It is best to do the jobs you don't like or those that are particularly difficult first. Otherwise, they won't get done or you will waste a lot of energy worrying about doing them, making you irritable and even depressed.

To-do lists mean that you can enjoy your relaxation time more since you are not trying to relax while your brain is still worrying over that day's chores. It will also help you to sleep better—which, in turn, will give you more energy.

Don't be afraid to reshuffle your lists. If you don't manage to get something done, move it to

QUICK ENERGY BOOSTERS

Add a method of relaxation to your to-do list for every day—you are much more likely to actually do it if you have scheduled it. Choose a massage, aromatherapy bath, meditation, or a short walk.

another day. The lists are there to take the stress off, not to add more.

A typical to-do list

Work:

All week—Start in-house magazine, decide topics and structure

Monday—Call suppliers and see if they want to advertise in magazine

Tuesday—Determine price of printing and mailing

Wednesday—Organize open days

Thursday and Friday—Open

Home:

Monday—Organize baby-sitting for anniversary

Tuesday—Buy diapers

Tuesday—Buy lightbulb for hall

Friday—Get money for cleaners and baby-sitter

Saturday—Go through baby clothes and put away ones that are too small

Saturday—Do laundry

Personal:

Sunday—Wedding

Monday and Friday—Exercise at gym

Tuesday—Dance class

Wednesday—Yoga

Thursday—Anniversary dinner

Friday—Pick up friends at airport

CONSERVE YOUR ENERGY

● Get your partner (and kids if you have any) to help with chores around the house. If you can afford it, get some help from a cleaner.

● If you are always running around doing things for other people but find at the end of the day you are exhausted, with no time left to do anything for yourself, you should learn to say "no" when you are asked to do yet another favor.

● Cut down on going to places or events that you really don't want to go to; only go if you really want to and if you have the energy.

● At work and at home, learn to delegate, especially at very busy times. This will help to get the job done and will allow you to conserve your energy so that whatever you do yourself is done efficiently. Don't fall into the trap of thinking that the job isn't done properly unless you do it yourself; eventually, you will collapse with exhaustion and nothing will get done at all.

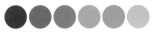
Nutrition and diet

Food is like fuel for the body. If you put poor-quality or no food into your body, like a car with the wrong or poor-quality gasoline, it won't function as it should, and eventually it won't run at all.

Poor diet and fatigue can very easily become a vicious cycle. A poor diet makes you feel more tired. When you are tired, shopping for food and cooking become yet more chores that have to be done, snack meals and stimulants become more appealing (chocolate, cakes, coffee, and tea), more vitamin deficiencies occur, and you end up feeling more tired than ever.

If you are lacking in energy, ask yourself if you are under- or overeating, missing meals, eating enough protein and fiber, drinking enough water, drinking too much alcohol, eating lots of sugary foods, and getting enough vitamins and minerals.

A good diet for making sure you have enough energy is one that includes:

- Fish (especially oily fish such as sardines and herring)
- Freshly made soups
- Chicken
- Farm eggs three times a week
- Lots of vegetables, especially green leafy ones such as spinach
- Salads
- Fresh fruit
- Lots of legumes
- Nuts and seeds
- Granola and oats
- Soybeans, tofu, miso paste (in soups)
- Vegetable oils (such as olive and grapeseed)
- Only a few dairy products (and none if you are damp—see p. 63— or have a cold)
- No sugar
- Plenty of yang foods (e.g., brown rice, whole-grain cereals, root vegetables, fish, legumes, and lentils)—see p. 63
- Lots of water, filtered if possible

All foods should be organic wherever possible, and alcohol should be avoided altogether since it is a depressant (it makes your sugar levels fluctuate, which can make you feel tired). Avoid coffee (even decaffeinated), and be careful with tea, which can overstimulate the adrenals. Herbal teas are best, and chamomile, peppermint, verbena, and lemon are all great for relaxing the nervous system. Dandelion, nettle, sage, and rosehip teas all help support the liver and help with detoxing.

If you are undereating or missing meals because you don't have enough time to prepare them, you can always fall back on eggs, cheese, salads, and soup, all of which are quick and easy to prepare, yet still supply you with the necessary vitamins and minerals to satisfy your energy requirements.

HOW TO EAT FOR ENERGY

Sometimes it is not what you are eating that is the problem but *how* you are eating it.

Here is a list of things to help you get the most from your food:

- Do not sit down to eat if you are upset or angry, as this will prevent you from digesting your food properly.

- Try to give yourself time to relax after work before eating dinner.

- Don't eat quickly and try not to overeat.

- Don't eat a heavy meal before going to sleep.

- It is better not to drink while eating because liquid dilutes the digestive enzymes.

- Always sit down to eat and try to concentrate on enjoying your food—its taste, smell, and colors.

- Eat three small to medium meals a day and two to three snacks.

- Don't go more than two and a half hours without food.

- Eat a big breakfast, since you haven't eaten anything for about twelve hours and your blood sugar levels will be low.

- Between-meal snacks should be rich in vitamins, minerals, and antioxidants. Fruit, either fresh or dried, and nuts and seeds are great snacks.

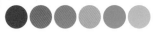
Cooking The way you cook your food is also important; some cooking methods can help to preserve nutrients, while others do the opposite. Here are some guidelines for healthy cooking:

- Remember that vitamins and minerals can be lost in the cooking process, especially Vitamins B and C, which are water-soluble. When you cook vegetables it is best to steam rather than boil them (if you boil them, many of the vitamins are leached into the water). If you must boil your vegetables, at least save the water for broth, or drink it—it is rich in nutrients.
- Fry as little as possible (although stir-frying is fine).
- Brush vegetables clean and scrape them rather than peel them; the skin is full of vitamins and minerals.
- Vitamin C is killed when exposed to the air, so eat your fruit and vegetables fresh and prepare them just before cooking.

CAFFEINE

Caffeine is found in coffee, tea, cocoa, chocolate, cola, and other carbonated drinks. It affects the nervous system, the heart, and blood circulation, and gives us a fake energy boost. It also acts like a drug. The more you consume, the more you need to be able to feel its effects until eventually you will have to ingest huge amounts of caffeine just to get a slight energy boost.

Tea is not as bad as coffee, but cutting them both out is preferable. Soft drinks with caffeine are even worse than coffee and tea because they also contain lots of sugar or artificial sweeteners. Too much of these can give you "the sugar blues," making you feel low and depressed: The body responds to a sudden influx of sugar into the bloodstream by producing insulin, which lowers the blood sugar level, leaving you drowsy, irritable, and unable to concentrate.

Note: Caffeine can cancel the effects of homeopathic medication for up to sixty days afterward.

Balancing your diet To maintain your health, have enough energy, and be able to fight off disease, you need a balanced diet that includes all five of the main nutrient groups (carbohydrate, protein, fat, fiber, and vitamins and minerals) in the correct proportions, along with plenty of water.

Carbohydrates are made up of carbon, hydrogen, and oxygen, and produce energy when their carbon molecules bind with oxygen in the bloodstream. They supply the body with instant energy and should therefore make up about fifty to sixty percent of our diet.

Carbohydrates are either starches or sugars, but we should mainly eat those that are starches, such as plant-based foods (cereals, bread, legumes, and root vegetables). As with all foods, it is better to eat them in their natural form (or as natural as possible) rather than refined. Fruit contains sugary carbohydrates; so do vegetables, but in much smaller quantities. Refined carbohydrates such as cake, cookies, and candy provide instant energy, which is fine in an emergency, but it won't sustain us over long periods of time. Starchy carbohydrates, on the other hand, take two hours to be used and absorbed, providing you with energy throughout the day. So for constant energy, it is best to eat starchy carbohydrates at the majority of your meals, with only a small intake of sugary carbohydrates for short bursts of energy. Beware of eating too many carbohydrates, however. If you eat more than you need for energy, the excess carbohydrate will be converted into fat and stored.

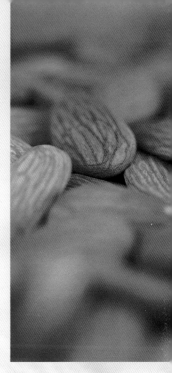

Protein The body needs protein to build muscle, repair tissue, maintain cells, and regulate bodily functions. We need protein for energy, and if we don't eat enough, we feel tired, irritable, and unable to concentrate. Between ten and fifteen percent of your food intake should be protein, depending upon how much you exercise and how much muscle you have.

There are twenty-two amino acids in proteins. Different foods contain different combinations of them, so you need to eat a variety of proteins to get all of them.

Protein foods include meats, legumes, dairy products, cheese, eggs, fish, poultry, nuts, seeds, whole-wheat bread, beans, and tofu. Some starchy foods like potatoes, white bread, and pasta also contain moderate amounts of protein.

If you eat more protein than you need for building muscle, your body will use it for energy by converting it to glucose. However, if you don't use this energy, it will be converted to fat and stored. Because protein takes longer than carbohydrates to be used by the body, it is good for giving you energy over long periods of time and for helping to control blood sugar levels.

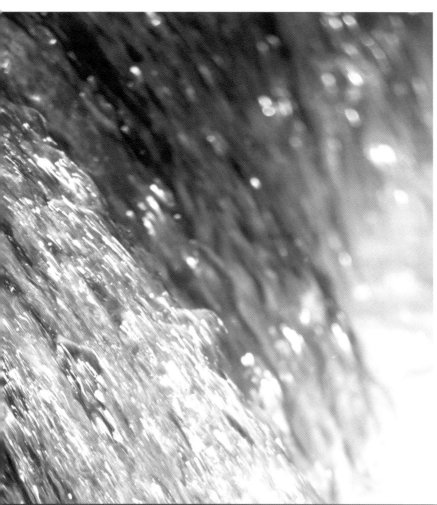

Fat The food industry promotes low-fat food because people who are conscious of putting on weight are prepared to pay more for them, even though many of them are full of sugars and additives. Not all fats are bad for you, but it is important to eat the right kinds.

There are three types of fat: polyunsaturated, monosaturated, and saturated. Fat is found in lots of foods and is the slowest food group to be converted to glucose and used as energy, so it is good for providing longer-term energy. Be careful, though, because as with proteins and carbohydrates, the energy that is not used is stored as body fat. Fat also helps vitamins A and D, which are fat-soluble, to be carried into the bloodstream and absorbed. A mixture of all three fats should make up thirty percent of your diet.

Saturated fat is found mainly in dairy foods, eggs, meat, and processed foods such as pies, cakes, cookies, and pastries. Polyunsaturated fat is found mainly in plant oils, including corn, safflower, sunflower, and nut and seed oils. They contain essential fatty acids (EFAs), linoleic acid, and alpha-linoleic acid, all of which are important for a healthy immune system, for energy conversion, and for keeping you well. If you are low in EFAs, as most people are, you will suffer from low levels of energy. Fatty acids, EPA, and DHA are found in oily fish.

Monosaturated fat is found mainly in olives, olive oil, canola oil, peanut oil, plant oils, nuts, seeds, and avocados. They are high in vitamin E, which is an antioxidant.

Fiber Lack of fiber in the diet can be a cause of sluggishness and low energy, as well as headaches and constipation. There are two types of fiber: insoluble and soluble. Insoluble fiber is found mainly in whole wheat, corn, brown rice, vegetables, and legumes. They help speed up the elimination of waste, which is good for your energy levels because it prevents constipation and the bloated, sluggish feeling that can accompany it. Soluble fiber is found mainly in legumes, oats, rye, apples, and citrus and other fruits. All types of fiber help regulate blood sugar levels, keep a constant flow of energy, and prevent hunger.

Alcohol Excess alcohol is damaging to many bodily functions and can reduce energy levels by disrupting sleep and blood sugar levels.

Water is vital for life and energy; if you don't drink enough, you can become dehydrated, making you feel weak, dizzy, faint, and eventually very unwell. Water plays a part in almost all bodily functions. It transports nutrients to and from cells, and is also very important for circulation, digestion, and excretion. Water also helps with regulating body temperature.

Most of us don't drink nearly enough water. Drinking about eight glasses a day should help to

CLEANSING DIET

Cleansing your body will make you feel more energized, especially if you have been eating too much of the wrong foods. You should eat lots of fresh fruit and vegetables, and drink lots of water to aid detoxification. You can also drink herbal teas.

improve energy and give a healthy glow to the skin. Filtered water is preferable, and a glass of water in the morning with lemon helps balance your energy.

Macrobiotics The theory of macrobiotics holds that the more "living" foods we put into our bodies, the more alive we will actually feel. Living foods are fresh foods that still have life in them and do not have colors, additives, emulsifiers, preservatives, and stabilizers added to them.

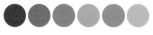 the **e n e r g y** plan

Vegetables, fruit, nuts, seeds, and legumes are all living foods. They are also easy to digest and provide vitamins, minerals, and fiber.

Macrobiotics, like Chinese medicine, looks at the energy of food in terms of yin and yang. If we eat too many yang/heating foods, we will feel restless, overreactive, and unable to relax, and have difficulty sleeping, almost as if we have too much energy. This is especially true if one is already a "hot" person, i.e., someone who feels hot, has a red complexion, is often restless, and walks and talks quickly.

On the other hand, too many yin/cooling foods will make us feel listless, lacking in energy, even depressed. Again this is especially true if we are already a "cold" person, i.e., someone who feels cold, is usually quiet, walks and talks slowly, and is often tired. See p. 63 for lists of "warming" and "cooling" foods.

Food and culture/religion Some cultures believe that food is not just fuel to fill our bodies, but that many food-related illnesses are due to a lack of spiritual connection with the food we eat. Almost all religions and spiritual traditions

ENERGY DIET FOR TRAVEL

When you are traveling, your diet should consist of one type of food, as far as is possible. This diet has proven to be very successful for many politicians, who need to be fully alert on arrival at their destination in order to participate in important meetings or international conferences:

● Eat one kind of food, preferably protein, throughout the twenty-four hours, from when you wake up on the day of travel (eggs, fish, low-fat cheese, meat, poultry, nuts, seeds), plus three to five portions of fruit throughout the day. Add more fruit if desired.

● Drink a minimum of eight 6-ounce glasses of water throughout the twenty-four hours, and no alcohol until arrival. If jet lag is to be avoided, no alcohol should be consumed, even after arrival. The following morning, your regular diet of complex carbohydrates, fat, and protein (see p. 89) should be resumed as usual.

POWER FOODS

Make sure you eat at least one power food every day. Here are some of them:

- Avocado: a great food for helping to increase your energy. It is a good source of B vitamins, and contains monosaturated fat, which protects against heart disease, and vitamin E, which is an antioxidant and great for your skin and circulation. Avocado is also a good source of copper, which helps red blood cell development and the absorption of iron from other foods. It also contains fiber.
- Bananas: a good source of fiber that beneficial bacteria crave, full of vitamin B6, good for digestion, and rich in potassium, which helps with high blood pressure. Because bananas are naturally high in carbohydrate, they give you piles of energy.
- Citrus fruits: help with energy levels because they are a powerful antioxidant and good for the immune system. They are also vital for the formation of collagen and connective tissue in the skin and blood vessels, which is important if you are training or doing vigorous activities. They are a good source of folic acid, which helps to produce red blood cells to carry oxygen around the body which, in turn, is vital for your energy.

regard food as sacred, and the eating of it is a sacred act (including Native Americans, Jews, Christians, Hindus, and Muslims).

Ayurvedic medicine teaches that food should not only taste good, but it should also appeal to all the other senses as well. It is therefore necessary to make sure you like the look of your plate and table before you eat and enjoy the smell of the food you choose to eat. Even finding foods that

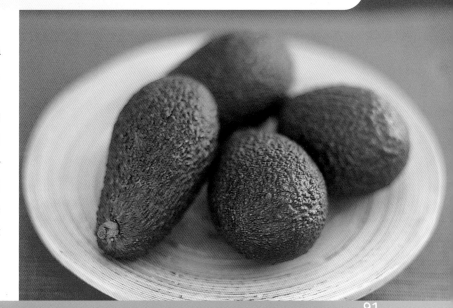

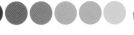

you like the sound of is encouraged, as well as those whose texture feels good to you.

Many religions and New Age followers believe that food should be prepared with love. For example, if you are making soup, say a prayer for everyone who is going to eat it, imagining that you are making a magical broth with healing powers to increase everyone's energy.

Foods for balancing blood-sugar levels Fluctuating blood-sugar levels are a common cause of low energy. If your blood sugar is low (hypoglycemia), you may feel tired and/or dizzy, be unable to concentrate, and have a craving for sweet foods. Low blood sugar can be caused by missing meals, taking prolonged exercise without any sustenance, or by a diet that is high in sugar or alcohol. The body responds to these stimuli by releasing extra insulin, which may make blood-sugar levels dip too low. Many women experience low blood sugar before their periods. Chromium deficiency is said to be a cause of low blood sugar, so it is a good idea to eat lots of foods containing chromium, such as shellfish, cheese, whole grains, and legumes. Caffeine should be avoided, as it can worsen the problem of fluctuating blood-sugar levels.

Meals consisting of whole foods and a combination of carbohydrates, proteins, and fat at each meal should be taken regularly. Plenty of low-glycemic foods in every meal will help maintain blood glucose levels and provide energy throughout the day. It will also help with hunger pangs. Fat and protein are low-glycemic foods, so a little of each should be included in every meal.

Other suitable foods are legumes, lentils, chickpeas, soybeans, baked beans, kidney beans, butter beans, barley, apples, dried apricots, peaches, plums, cherries, grapefuit, avocado, zucchini, spinach, peppers, onions, mushrooms, leafy greens, leeks, green beans, sprouts, snow peas, cauliflower, broccoli, natural yogurt, milk, and peanuts.

Note: The worst thing you can do if you suffer from low blood sugar is to reach for a sugary snack!

Allergies If you suffer from allergies, lots of whole, unprocessed, and most importantly, organic foods are best. If you have a wheat or gluten allergy, try millet, rice, and corn (polenta), buckwheat, and corn or rice pastas. Soy and rice milk are good alternatives to cow's milk for anyone who is intolerant to lactose.

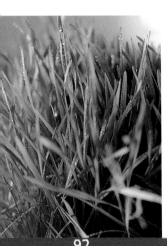

Vitamin and mineral supplements

Vitamin and mineral supplements help increase your energy by treating deficiencies. For example, if you have blood deficiency, supplements of iron and blue-green algae, along with a good-quality multivitamin and mineral supplement, will help to build the blood—and hence your energy—more quickly than if you try to do it with food alone.

Some people know that their diet is poor, and they take supplements so that they feel they are getting the nutrients that they need in spite of their bad eating habits. This is better than nothing, but is not a substitute for a healthy diet. Some believe that the quality of food and the soil in which it grows is so bad these days that no matter how healthy your diet is, you cannot possibly get the full range and quantity of nutrients needed.

Either way, you will certainly be short of energy if you neglect to make sure you are getting enough vitamins and minerals, either through your diet or with supplementation.

Below is a list of supplements that will help if you are feeling tired all the time or low in energy. You should be able to find most of them at good health food stores, where over-the-counter advice should also be available.

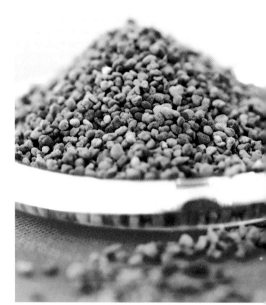

○ **Bee pollen:** dramatically increases energy.

DOSE: a few granules daily for three days, then slowly increase to two teaspoons daily.

Note: Some people can have an allergic reaction, so discontinue use if you develop a rash, wheezing, discomfort, or other allergic symptoms.

○ **Brewer's yeast:** a good source of vitamin B, which is vital for energy.

DOSE: one teaspoon daily, then work up to two teaspoons daily over a two-week period.

○ **Vitamin B complex:** crucial for supplying energy to the body. Most B-vitamins help our bodies convert food to energy and help maintain the nervous system. Deficiency of B-vitamins can result in fatigue. They are water soluble and cannot be stored in the body, so we have to make sure we get enough of them every day. Any excess will be passed out through the urine, making it bright yellow. It is better to take vitamin B complex rather than individual B-vitamins.

DOSE: 100 mg, three times daily with meals.

○ **Vitamin B1 (thiamine):** essential for growth, health of muscles and nerves, and the conversion of carbohydrates into energy. Signs of deficiency are: irritability, depression, loss of appetite, poor digestion, and dark shadows under the eyes. Vitamin B1 is found in meat, fish, beans, nuts, seafood, whole grains, legumes, potatoes, wheat germ, and yeast.

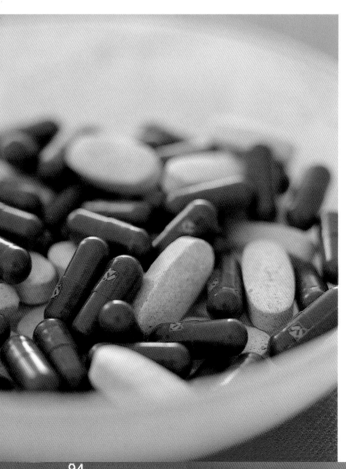

○ **Vitamin B2 (riboflavin):** extracts energy from proteins and carbohydrates. It is essential for growth, health of skin, eyes, and red blood cells. Signs of deficiency are: lack of stamina, feeling nervous all the time, and dry hair and skin. Vitamin B2 is found in meat, soybeans, eggs, vegetables, chicken, milk, cheese, and yeast.

○ **Vitamins B3 (niacin) and B6 (pyridoxine):** important for growth, health of the nervous system, helps counteract stress (and therefore helps energy), and important for the health of the skin. Signs of deficiency are: insomnia, irritability, anxiety, depression, headaches, and feeling shaky. They are found in lean meats, fish, whole grains, chicken, nuts, potatoes, bananas, dried fruit, and green vegetables.

○ **Folic acid:** essential for growth, blood, and fertility. Signs of deficiency are: fatigue, feeling weak, depression, and anemia. It is found in spinach, brussels sprouts, broccoli, potatoes, whole-wheat flour, and lentils.

○ **Vitamin B5 (pantothenic acid):** converts energy from proteins, fats, and carbohydrates. Signs of deficiency are: dry skin and hair, fatigue. It is found in eggs, liver, meat, nuts, whole grains, and yeast.

○ **Vitamin B12:** fights fatigue and helps to prevent anemia; important for the health of the nerves, blood, and skin. Signs of deficiency are: fatigue and anemia. It is found in liver, chicken, lean meat, eggs, yeast, milk, and cheese.

Vitmain B12 is not found in vegetables, so it is very important for strict vegans to take B12 supplements (2,000 mcg daily).

○ **Vitamin C:** increases energy and helps prevent disease, aids recovery from illness, combats stress, and helps in the body's absorption of iron. Signs of deficiency are: regular colds, bleeding gums, susceptibility to bruising, fatigue, frequent infections. Found in fresh fruit (especially citrus), strawberries, rose hips, and vegetables—especially green, leafy ones.
DOSE: 3,000-8,000 mg daily.

○ **Minerals:** present in the soil and absorbed by plants. We get our minerals by eating either plants or animals that have eaten plants. For optimum health, energy, and vitality, we need more than fifteen different minerals, including iron, calcium, phosphorus, sodium, magnesium, potassium, and sulfur. Without them we develop symptoms of deficiency such as fatigue, depression, emotional tension, and anemia. Of all the minerals, a lack of iron and calcium are most commonly associated with energy loss.

○ **Iron:** deficiency is very common, especially in women. Iron deficiency starves the cells of oxygen, causing fatigue, irritability, and/or depression.

It is found in meat, liver, kidneys, whole-grain cereals, spinach, lentils, dried apricots, prunes, and peanut butter.
DOSE: as directed on the bottle.
NOTE: Do not take iron if you have a bacterial infection, since it can feed the bacteria.

○ **Calcium:** deficiency upsets the function of the nerves and muscles, causing excitability and inability to relax or sleep. It is found in dairy foods, fish, vegetables, and eggs.
DOSE: as directed on the bottle.

○ **Royal jelly:** the food supplied to the queen bee by the worker bees. It is taken from bee larvae and provides the queen with an amazing amount of energy and stamina, enabling her to produce, in twenty-four hours, an amount of eggs equal to two thousand times her body weight. She also lives five times longer than her workers. Research on royal jelly suggests that it is a great energizer because it contains protein, B vitamins, amino

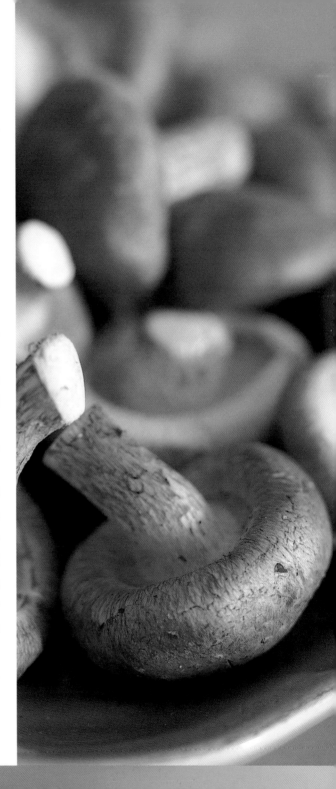

acids, and enzymes. Not only does it increase your energy, vitality, and stamina, but it also boosts the immune system and improves skin, nails, and hair. The Japanese believe that it helps old people recover their zest for life.

DOSE: two capsules, three times a day.

○ **Shiitake/reishi mushrooms:** help to build immunity and boost energy levels

DOSE: as directed on the label.

○ **Spirulina:** an excellent protein source and full of all the essential vitamins and minerals.

DOSE: between one and four pills, three times a day (if you get loose stools, start more slowly and build up).

○ **Ginseng:** known as "the root of life." Chinese doctors prescribe it for loss of vigor, anemia, nervous disorders, insomnia, and even as a sexual potency remedy. Even though it can help insomnia, it should not be taken late in the day because it is such a potent energizer that it could actually prevent you from sleeping. The Russians give ginseng to their astronauts to heighten their alertness, endurance, and energy. It is rich in nutrients, minerals, and trace elements.

DOSE: Consult a qualified herbalist for correct dose.

NOTE: Do not take at all during pregnancy.

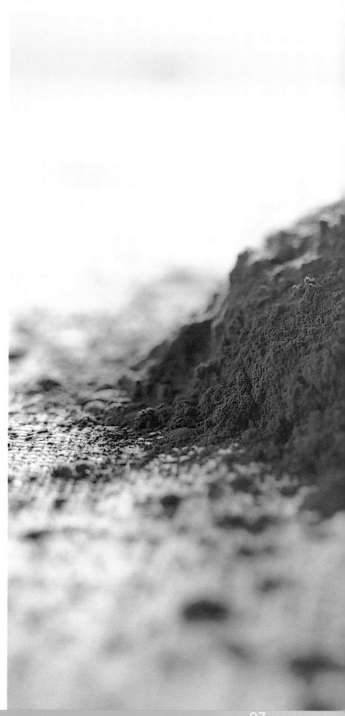

● **CoQ10 (coenzyme Q10, also known as "ubiquinone"):** a vitamin-like substance that helps the body convert food into energy. It can be found in food, and the body can make its own, but as we get older or become sick, we tend to make less.

DOSE: one to two 60-mg tablets with meals daily.

● **Blue-green algae:** a complete food source that contains all the vitamins and minerals we need to be healthy and full of vitality.

DOSE: one to four pills, three times daily (if you get loose stools or feel too excitable, take a lower dose and build up more slowly).

● **Wheatgrass:** can be made into a drink or taken in capsule form. It is rich in vitamins, minerals, and antioxidants.

DOSE: a half to one teaspoon daily.

NOTE: Always seek advice from a fully qualified and insured naturopath or nutritionist before taking any of the above if you are pregnant or suffering from any serious medical condition.

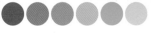
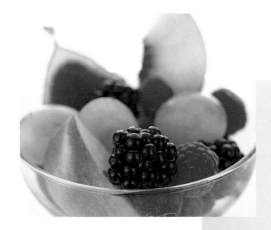

Your energy is your responsibility. What you choose to eat can determine how much or how little energy you have. If you choose to eat a high percentage of refined carbohydrates in your daily diet (i.e., white bread, pasta, pastries, candy bars, etc.) then your energy levels will be low. However, if you choose more complex carbohydrates (i.e., whole-grain bread, fresh fruit and vegetables, legumes, nuts and seeds) then your energy levels will be much higher. Acquiring and sustaining your energy levels can be that simple. It's about getting back to basics—naturally.

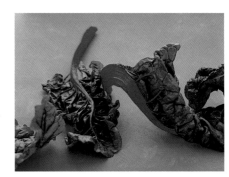

As the saying goes, "you are what you eat," but, more accurately, you are what you assimilate. Good digestion of food depends upon the quality of the food we eat. A varied and natural diet, preferably organic-based, provides the body with the nutrients it needs for optimum energy.

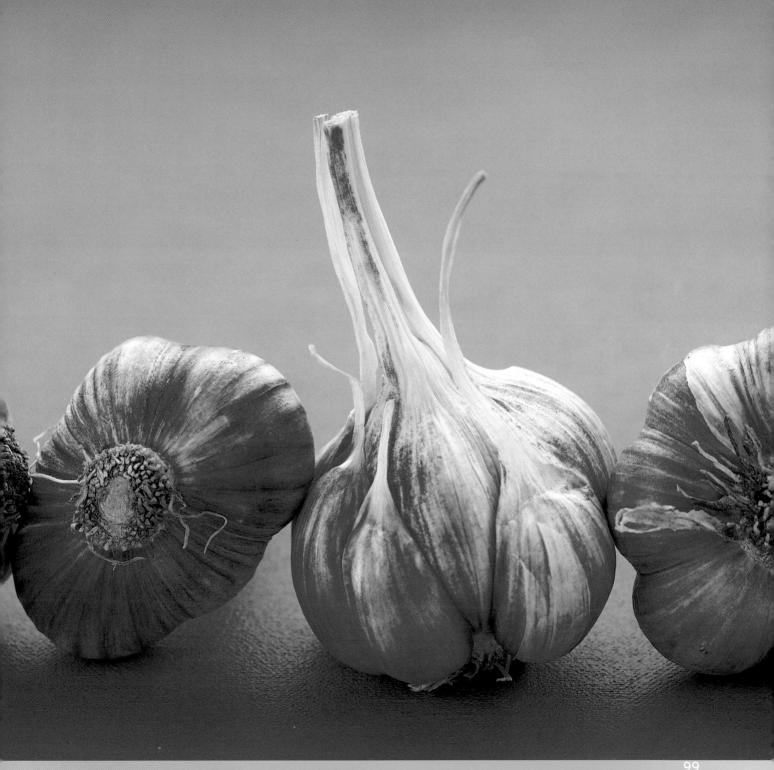

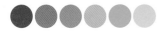

Exercise

One of the quickest ways to increase your energy levels is to move your body.

Staying in one position for too long for whatever reason is not healthy—it slows the body down, impairs circulation, makes the body hungry for oxygen, and stops energy from flowing, leaving you tired and lifeless.

Aerobic exercise increases the amount of air that you breathe into your lungs, giving the body

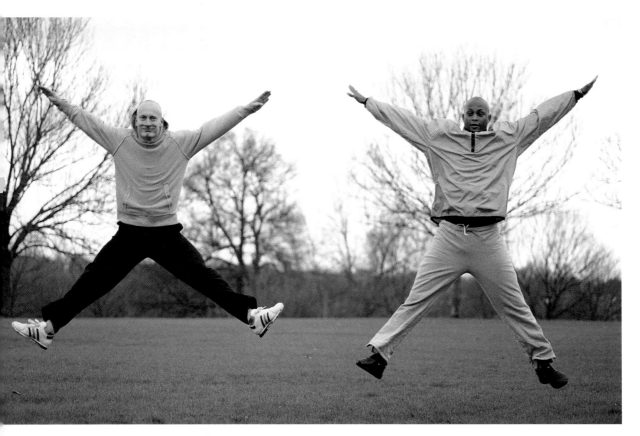

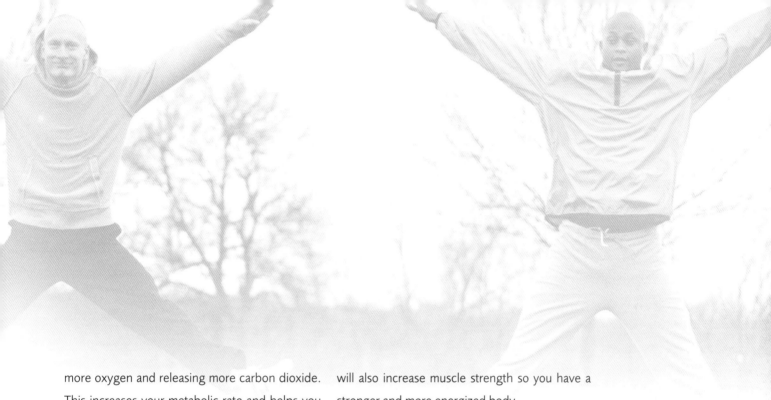

more oxygen and releasing more carbon dioxide. This increases your metabolic rate and helps you burn fuel/calories more quickly, thus giving you more energy. It also strengthens the lungs and heart so that oxygenated blood pumps around the body to every cell, muscle, and organ, which in turn makes you feel more alive and energetic. Just twenty minutes of aerobic exercise three or four times a week can make a world of difference to your energy levels. Choose between walking, swimming, rollerblading, cycling, squash, basketball, tennis, boxing, dancing, and horseriding. Exercising the major muscle groups increases the lean muscle tissue in your body. If you do strength training and aerobic exercise, you will also increase muscle strength so you have a stronger and more energized body.

Exercise improves flexibility and helps prevent osteoporosis. In addition to releasing tension in muscles, exercise releases endorphins and makes you feel happier. When you exercise, you also stimulate the lymph system and increase circulation, which helps you feel more energetic.

The exercises below include yoga, stretching, and qi gong. They will help you feel relaxed and become more flexible and energized. I have chosen them because I know that they are quite easy to do and will definitely start the ball rolling for increasing your energy. So, go for it! The more energy you use, the more energy you will get!

Note: It is important to rest for at least twenty-four hours between tougher aerobic exercise sessions (squash, basketball, etc.) in order to give the body time to recover. Walk on the days in between and do gentle stretching exercises (see pages 102–103).

Consult your doctor before doing any of the exercises in this book if you have had an illness, are pregnant or overweight, or you haven't exercised before or for a long time.

Warming up and cooling down

It is always very important to warm up before and cool down after any exercise so as to avoid any muscle aches or injuries.

BREATHING

Breathing

How we breathe is very closely connected to how we feel. When we are relaxed or asleep our breathing becomes slower, deeper, and more even, breathing from the diaphragm and stomach, not the chest. When we are frightened it is faster and more shallow, creating an imbalance of oxygen and carbon dioxide, which can make us feel light-headed and panicky. If you are constantly feeling stressed you may develop a habit of breathing in this way so that even when you are relaxing, you still feel stressed.

Correct breathing

1. Sit and relax.

2. Breathe deeply through your nose and let out a sigh.

3. Breathe in again, this time ensuring that you breathe into your chest, diaphragm, and stomach (until they expand), to the count of five.

4. Breathe out through your mouth from your stomach, diaphragm, and chest to the count of five.

You might find that the diaphragm doesn't expand as it should due to stiffness, but it will eventually become easier with practice. Find a few minutes throughout the day to take a break and practice your breathing.

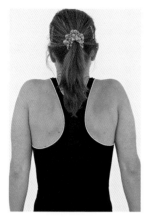

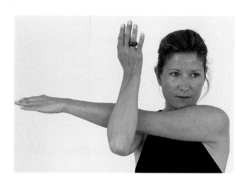

Warm-up and cool-down exercises

(All warm-up exercises should be held for a count of ten.)

1. Shrug your shoulders up and down a few times.

2. Turn your head from side to side and up and down.

3. Stretch your arms by lifting one arm up, bending it at the elbow, then letting your hand dangle behind your head. Repeat with the other arm.

4. Hold one arm straight out in front of you parallel to the floor and with the other hand move the arm toward the other side of your body until you feel a stretch in your upper arm. Repeat with the other arm.

5. Now, put one foot forward; with your heel on the floor, bend your other knee slightly and bend slightly forward—you should feel a stretch up the back of your leg. Repeat for the other leg.

6. With one hand holding onto a wall for balance, bend your left leg backward and hold your foot with your left hand. Repeat for the right leg. If you find this difficult, try it lying down on your side.

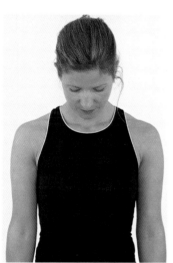

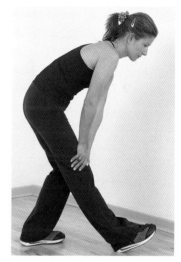

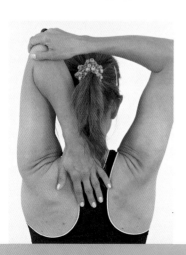

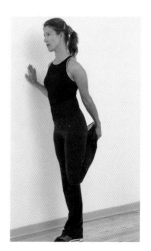

Walking

Of all the different types of exercise, walking is one of the easiest, as well as being inexpensive and very good for you.

In order to really benefit from walking you need to walk at a good pace, without stopping, for about twenty minutes. As you get fitter you need to increase the time and speed to reap the benefits. You should feel your lungs really working and breathe in more deeply than when at rest. However, you should be able to carry on a conversation with someone who is walking beside you.

Always wear suitable clothing and comfortable, supportive walking shoes. You should warm up for a few minutes before your walk by walking slowly, and gradually build up your speed and do the same at the end for cooling down. Be sure to stretch your legs before and after to prevent aches and pains (see p. 103).

The windmill routine

My grandfather lived to the age of ninety-one, was vibrant, active, and healthy right up until his last few months, and was an inspiration to all who knew him. He did the windmill exercise routine his whole life—wherever he went, whatever the weather. If you do nothing else in terms of exercise, at least try to do the windmill daily:

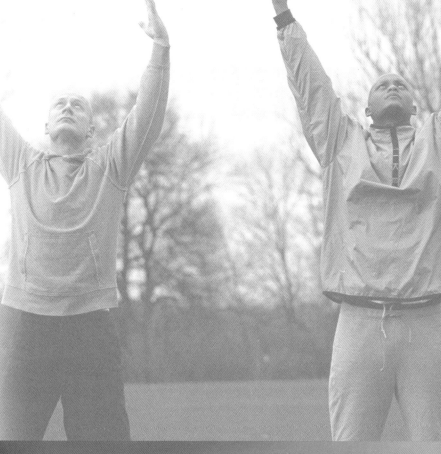

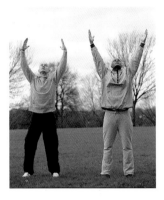

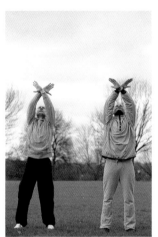

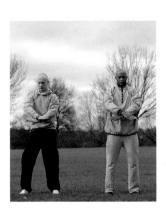

1. When you wake up in the morning, open the window and, no matter the weather, stand by the open window.

2. Take ten big, deep breaths of fresh air.

3. Put your arms up to the ceiling, with elbows just slightly bent, cross your hands above your head, and move them down to the side (like a windmill), still taking big, deep breaths.

4. Now bring both arms up from the side, cross them in front of your face and up above your head, then bring them down to the sides again, breathing deeply throughout. Repeat ten times.

5. Lift your arms above your head and take a big breath in.

6. Bend down with straight legs, reach for your toes, exhale slowly, and come up to a standing position. Repeat five times.

7. Now do ten jumping jacks, breathing deeply all the time.

8. Don't forget to close the window!

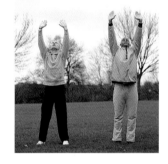

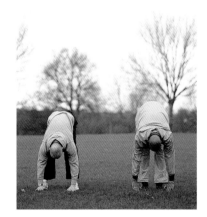

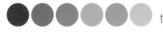

Strengthening exercises

Strengthening exercises should be done three times a week for about twenty to thirty minutes. Repeat fifteen times (one set) and increase as you begin to build strength. Work until the muscle begins to feel tired or shake slightly.

You will need an exercise band or ball, (see picture, page 107) or a set of free weights for some of the exercises.

Half push-ups for your chest (below)

1. Kneel down with your palms flat on the floor.

2. Bring the knees slightly backward.

3. Bend your elbows and, keeping your back straight, allow your upper body to dip toward the floor.

4. Try and go as low as possible, then slowly raise yourself back up again. Try to add a few more repetitions each week.

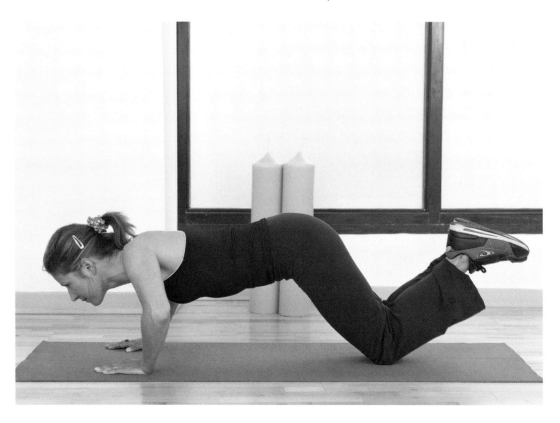

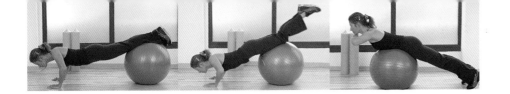

If you find the half push-ups too difficult, try using an exercise ball (above):

1. Lie on the exercise ball and get it into position with your thighs resting on it and your feet raised.

2. Put your hands on the floor and lower your body down between your hands, with a straight back. Slowly raise yourself back up again.

3. For a full push-up, rest your shins on the ball and continue as above.

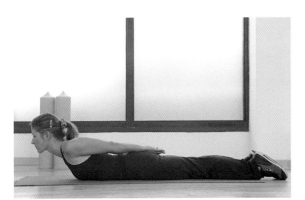

Back strengthener (above)

1. Lie on your stomach, with your hands behind your back or under your chin.

2. Keep your legs and hips on the floor and raise your upper body a few inches from the floor or as far as you can go. Don't look up.

If you find this too difficult, try using an exercise ball (see top right).

Bicep curl (right)

1. Stand on your elastic band, with your feet hip-width apart.

2. Bend your knees, slightly tuck in your stomach and bottom.

3. Hold the band in one hand with your arms by your side and slowly raise and bend your arm until your hand comes up to your shoulder.

4. Gently lower back to your side again.

5. Repeat for the other side.

Lateral raise (below)

1. Put the band in your right hand with your arm by your side.

2. With your feet hip-width apart and your

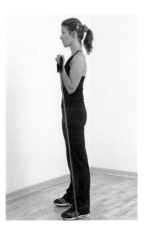

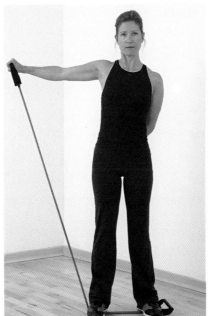

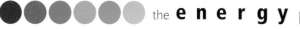

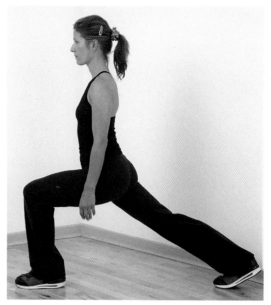

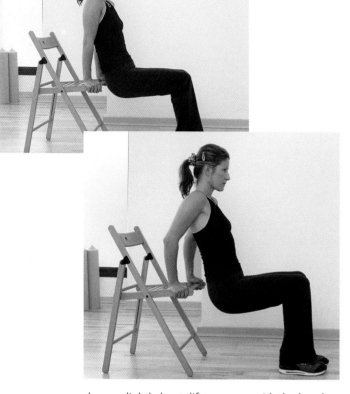

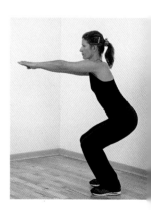

knees slightly bent, lift your arm with the band out to the side until your arm is parallel to the floor, then slowly lower your arm to the floor.

3. Repeat on the other side.

Tricep dips (above)

1. Sit on the edge of a sturdy chair.

2. With your hands holding the edge of the chair, lower yourself off the chair until your

elbows are at right angles to the floor.

3. Pull yourself back up, without sitting down.

4. Repeat.

Lunge (above)

1. Stand with feet hip-width apart and with your arms by your side.

2. Take a step forward with one leg and then bend both legs until the front leg is at right angles to the floor.

3. Come back to the starting position and repeat with the other leg.

Squat (right)

1. Stand with feet hip-width apart and arms out in front, parallel to the floor.

2. Squat down, keeping your back straight.

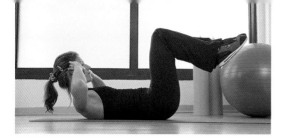

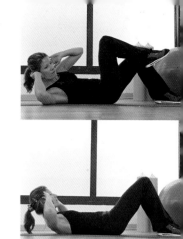

Keep your knees in line with your feet. Try and get your thighs parallel to the floor.

3. Slowly return to starting position and repeat.

Crunch (above)

1. Lie on your back, with your knees bent and your feet firmly on the floor.

2. With your hands at your temples, breathe out and raise your head and neck off the floor.

Slowly go back, but without touching the floor.

3. Repeat.

Side crunch (right)

1. Like the crunch, but this time raise one knee in toward the head and neck.

2. Put the knee back down, then raise the other knee in while raising your head and neck.

3 Raise both knees. Repeat all three parts of the exercise each time.

EXERCISE WHEN YOU'RE TRAVELING

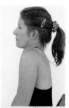

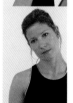

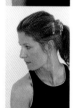

After traveling it is important to do some form of exercise to keep the blood and oxygen flowing to the muscles and brain and to help your body and mind adjust to any differences in time, food, weather, and culture.

Normal energy levels can plummet and may not return to normal as quickly as usual, even after rest. If this happens, be patient and listen to your body and mind. If your metabolism has slowed down and become sluggish, it might take more time than you would expect for the coordination of your body and mind to return to its normal patterns, especially after crossing time zones.

Listen to what your body is telling you. Try gentle, exploratory stretching exercises to bring your mind/body connection together again in a quiet "one-to-one" way—your body and yourself—and develop your routine slowly, possibly to include the following:

- Simple rolling of shoulders backward and forward
- Tilting neck toward one shoulder, then the other, looking over one shoulder and then the other
- Rotating ankles around in both directions and up and down with toes; also move heels up and down
- Shrugging shoulders up and down toward ears

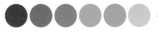

Chinese wisdom

The Chinese believe in balancing the flow of energy, or qi, around the body.

They believe that the qi can become blocked due to factors such as stress, shock, toxins, and emotional problems such as anger or grief, causing disease and disharmony. The ancient Chinese mapped out channels, or meridians, through which qi flows and used pressure and needles on precise points along these meridians to stimulate or regulate the qi's flow, thus increasing energy, lifting mood, and helping to treat specific illnesses. As well as working on these specific points, they also used medicines and exercises to remove blockages.

Qi gong

One exercise that helps to move the qi and build it is known as *qi gong,* which has been practiced in China for thousands of years. The term "qi gong" means "energy practice." It is a combination of breathing, posture, and meditation, and like yoga, it focuses our energy inward. It is often translated as "working with life energy." It is a precise routine that finds energy imbalances and corrects them. It helps to increase energy flow and emotional stability, promotes clear thinking, physical fitness, good health, and spiritual well-being.

Everyone can do qi gong; you can even perform it sitting down. Ideally it should be practiced every day and in doing so, you will notice a dramatic change in your energy levels.

Below are a few qi gong exercises that are easy to do and can increase your energy and vitality.

Holding the dantien

The dantien is about an inch below the navel and is where the qi is stored. It helps in lymphatic drainage and aids proper circulation.

1. Men should place their right hand on the dantien and the left hand over the right. Women should place their left hand on the dantien and the right hand over their left.

2. Relax your whole body, straighten your legs (but don't lock them), and concentrate on and breathe into the dantien.

3. Bend your knees and breathe out.

4. Repeat for a few minutes.

You can do this exercise for longer when you get used to it and you have the time.

Vital energy

Many people spend so much of their life running around that they forget what it feels like to be aware of their vital energy. Vital energy is always there, but we often tend to be so busy that we ignore it. Here is an exercise to help you reconnect and feel your own energy again. Most people feel a tingling sensation throughout their body after doing this exercise.

1. Stand with your shoes off, your feet hip-width apart, and your knees slightly bent.

2. Let your hands fall by your sides.

3. Imagine there is a rope from the top of your head to the sky, holding you upright.

4. Relax your shoulders and neck.

5. Close your eyes and become aware of your breathing.

6. Just stand and breathe for a few minutes.

7. Become aware of the center of your body, the area around your navel (your dantien). Breathe big, deep breaths into this area.

8. Focus on the dantien being the center of yourself and keep breathing slowly and steadily.

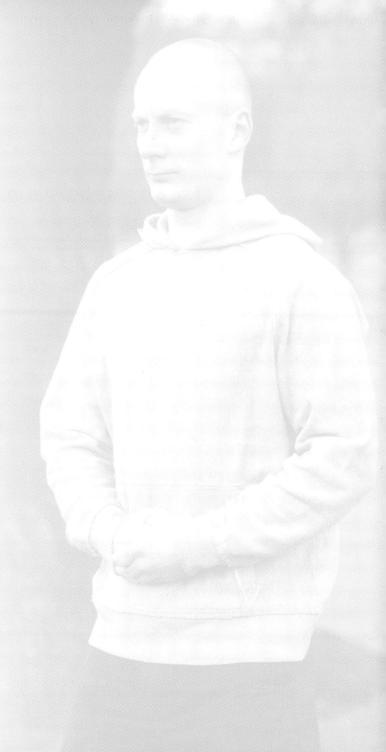

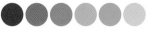
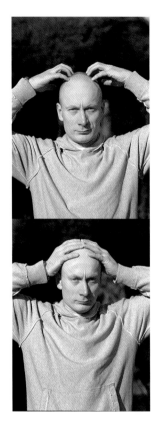

Qi gong slap

Do this exercise every morning when you wake up to start your day with a boost of energy.

1. Tap your head with your fingertips and gently pat your head all over with your hands. Then stroke your hair, neck, and shoulders.

2. Pat your hands down the inside of each arm (one at a time), starting at the armpit and making your way down to your fingertips.

3. Now pat up the outside of each arm (one at a time) from your fingertips up to your shoulders.

4. Gently tap and pat your upper chest, down your sternum, and around to your hips.

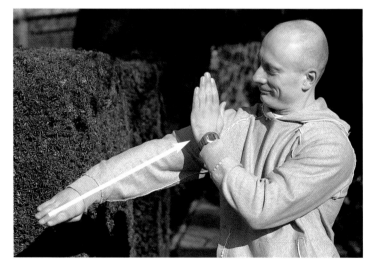

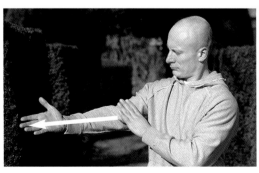

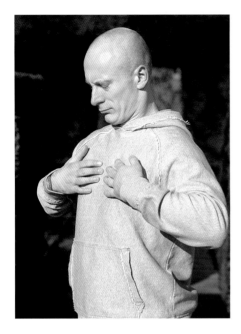

5. Pat your hips and down the outside of both legs, then brush your feet.

6. Continue patting up the insides of both legs, around to the back.

7. Pat the lower back—this is very good for the kidneys.

8. Repeat the whole exercise ten times. On the tenth time, let your hands rest on the kidneys for a minute, then circle your hands around to your stomach and let your hands settle (for a minute), one hand over the other, just under your belly button.

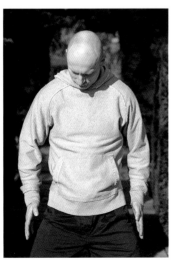

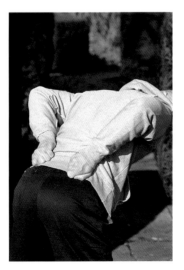

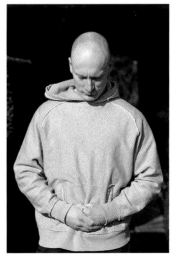

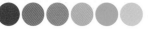

Balancing the energy

Our bodies are often out of alignment. There are all sorts of things that can throw our bodies out, such as always sleeping on one side, working at a computer at an awkward angle or without taking breaks, carrying a bag on one side, and standing with more weight on one leg than the other. I remember experiencing neck and shoulder pain after having a baby, and eventually realized it stemmed from the way I was looking down at her lovingly while breast-feeding. Here is an exercise that can improve the body's symmetry, allowing the energy to flow more smoothly around it.

1. Stand with your feet hip-width apart and your knees slightly bent.

2. Spread your arms out to the sides as if hugging a massive ball.

3. Imagine the ball is full of energy, then pull your hands into your chest, bringing all the energy into you.

4. Let your chin drop to your chest.

5. Repeat the whole exercise ten times.

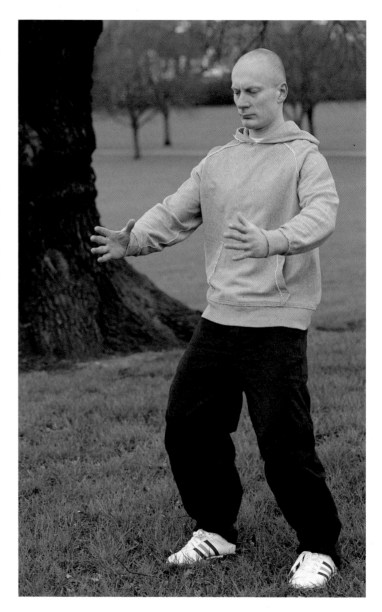

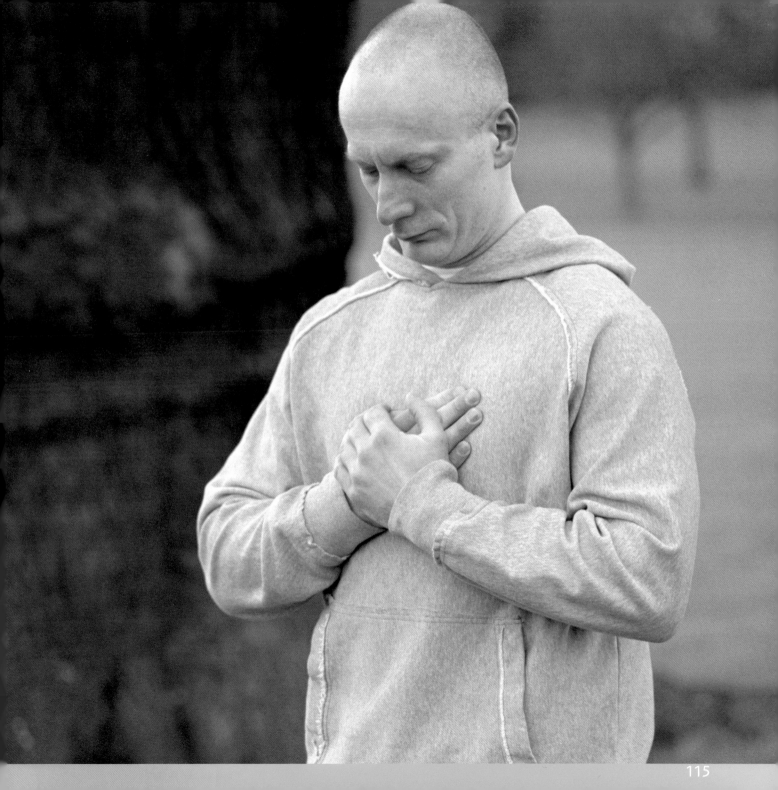

Qi gong tree

According to the theory of qi gong, every time we place our bare feet on the ground when we walk, we reconnect with the earth's vital energy.

1. Stand with your feet hip-width apart, stretch out your toes, and bend your knees slightly.

2. Gently pull up your abdominal muscles while allowing your buttocks to sink toward the floor.

3. Drop your shoulders and allow your chin to drop slightly, relaxing your neck. You should feel your body grounded from the waist downward.

4. Imagine that your head is being held up by an imaginary rope.

5. Hang your arms, bent loosely by your sides, as if holding onto an imaginary ball. You should feel completely relaxed; if anything hurts, you should breathe it out.

6. Imagine you are a tree and your feet grow roots deep into the ground. As you breathe in, imagine that you are drawing up the earth's goodness through your roots to nourish you.

7. With each breath, positive energy is taken in, stimulating the flow of qi around the body.

8. With each breath out, all negative energy, toxins, and anxieties are exhaled into the earth.

9. You should feel like all your cares have been taken away. Your mind should feel peaceful.

The qi gong ball

This exercise helps to increase vitality at any time of the day. It increases the energy in the dantien, where energy is stored (see p. 110). After you have done this exercise you will probably feel a hot, tingling sensation in your hands.

1. Stand with your feet hip-width apart, your knees slightly bent, and your hands in front of your abdomen (dantien), with your palms facing inward.

2. Imagine that a ball of energy is coming from your abdomen (dantien) and filling your hands.

3. Slowly, move your hands apart so that you are holding the growing ball of energy in your palms.

4. Once the ball has grown to the size of a big beach ball, hold it for a few minutes.

5. Imagine that the ball of energy contracts when your hands move closer and expands when they are farther apart. Repeat several times, contracting and expanding the energy ball.

6. Now bring your palms back to your abdomen (dantien), letting the ball contract back into the abdomen until it just feels like a spark. Hold your hands there for a minute.

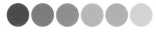

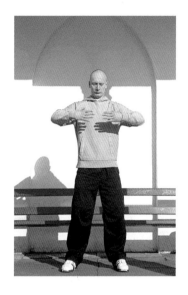

The energy sweep

This exercise stimulates the flow of energy in all the meridians, especially the gallbladder, large intestine, liver, kidneys, and spleen. Sweep as fast or as slow as you like and you will feel the energy starting to flow.

1. Stand with your feet hip-width apart and your knees slightly bent.

2. Lift your elbows up and bring your hands (palms facing inward) into your chest.

3. Stretch your arms out to the side and then up above your head.

4. Bend your arms and cradle the back of your head with your hands.

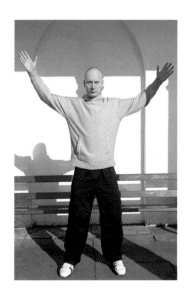

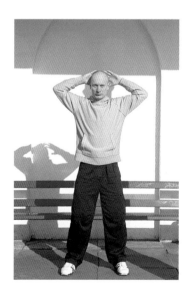

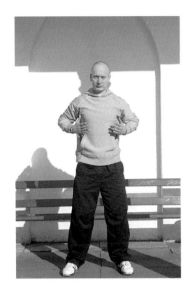

5. Sweep your hands down your neck, over your shoulders, down your chest, and rest your palms on your lower ribs.

6. Sweep around to your back and rest one palm over each kidney.

7. Sweep your palms over your hips and down the outside of your legs.

8. Sweep over the feet and up the insides of your legs.

9. Rest one hand over the other, just under your belly button.

10. Repeat ten to twenty times.

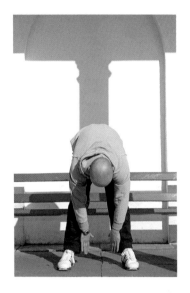

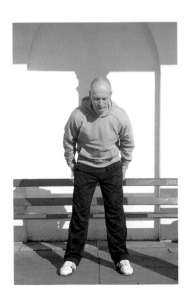

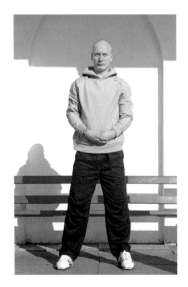

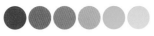

Yoga

Yoga originated in India about 5,000 years ago and is known for its ability to help you relax deeply, both mentally and physically.

The yoga most often practiced in the West is hatha yoga (although there are many other types), which concentrates on postures (*asanas*) that stretch, realign, and balance the body, and breathing (*pranayama*) that helps you to relax and center your mind and body. It can also include meditation (*dhyana*), which helps to calm and focus. The result is a relaxed, centered, and well-balanced body with a focused and refreshed mind.

Yoga helps to bring balance into your life. The word *yoga* means "union," meaning the balance between mind, body, and spirit. It is about bringing together the balance of your physical, mental, and spiritual states; for example, your state of mind will affect your immune system and hormonal systems, which will affect your circulation and breathing. So in order to treat physical fatigue, you need to look at your mental and spiritual needs, too.

Like many of the ancient traditional medicines, yoga holds that the key to good health and happiness lies in the free flow of energy (prana) around the body. Yogis believe that if we live in harmony with nature and keep our energy balanced by learning to control our breathing and our posture, we will be healthy. Yoga's precise postures work deep into the body, encouraging the blood to circulate and give you endless energy. The blood then nourishes every organ and softens all the muscles and ligament tissue. The deep stretching of yoga brings the bones and muscles back into alignment and also lubricates the joints, helping to keep you flexible even as you grow older.

Indian medicine believes that we take in vital energy through breathing. Our breathing also helps us get more oxygen and therefore helps with other functions such as digestion and concentration. Yoga helps you to use what you take in for energy. It will help you to store, direct, and control your energy, and also to balance your chakras so that your energy can flow properly.

In yoga a restless mind is compared to a chattering monkey. If you are very stressed, you will most likely end up with a head full of racing thoughts and suffer from anxiety and depression—all of which will deplete your energy. Practicing yoga will help to calm your mind and quiet the chattering monkey.

Yoga tones the body, delays aging, helps the joints and skeleton, and strengthens the circulation, as well as the heart and lungs. Therefore the blood receives more oxygen, breathing and digestion are improved, posture is enhanced, and the spine becomes more flexible. The nervous and hormonal systems are balanced, the body relaxes, organs and glands are nourished, chakras are balanced, and toxins are removed. And, of course, yoga gives you energy.

Breathing

There is a great yoga proverb that says, "Life is in the breath; he who only half breathes half lives." Breathing is an important medicine, without which we die. It helps to feed the brain and calms the nervous system, which has an effect on all the other physical systems of the body. Our lungs are our connection with the outside world. When we breathe in we take in new energy and life and when we exhale, we breathe out the old, the waste, and the expired. Buddhists believe that every breath in is a new life and every breath out a little death, so taking in deep, joyful breaths is a way of getting a dose of life and vitality.

Our breath becomes constricted because of trapped memories, experiences, and emotions such as fear, anger, anxiety, sadness, and grief. By using our breath we can slowly release these constrictions. Breathing techniques are some of the oldest, most effective, and easiest ways of stimulating and balancing energy within the body.

Yoga teaches breathing techniques to improve your energy, mind, mood, physical conditions, and immune system, and even help slow down the aging process.

Try not to be competitive when doing yoga. Go at your own pace and always come out of a posture very carefully. It's best to wear loose clothes for yoga, and you should not eat for two hours beforehand as the digestive process uses up energy.

Before doing any yoga you need to learn the breathing techniques on the following pages and, as with any other form of exercise, always start with a warm-up routine.

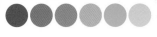

Breathing the yoga way (pranayama)

Pranayama is the yogic science of breathing. It is an excellent tool, as it encourages you to breathe deeply and fully, bringing oxygen deep into the cells and pulling out toxins. It also sends a surge of energy through every cell of your body.

1. Lie on your back and make yourself comfortable. Bring your feet close up to your buttocks, with the soles of your feet together, and allow the knees to fall apart with your hands gently resting on your abdomen. This posture stretches the lower abdomen, which enhances the breathing practice. (If you find this position difficult, just lie on your back with your hands on your abdomen; with each inhalation lift your arms out and up above your head, and with each exhalation bring your arms back to your sides.)

2. Breathe in through your nose and feel your abdomen expand and contract.

3. Breathe out through your nose and notice your abdomen flatten.

4. If you feel comfortable you can extend the inhalation of the breath so it comes up from the abdomen into the chest, allowing you to breathe in longer and deeper.

5. Bring your knees back together and stretch out your legs.

6. Repeat five to ten times.

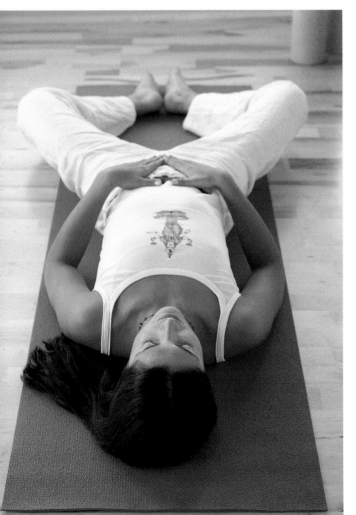

Alternate-nostril breathing

Alternate-nostril breathing stimulates both sides of the brain and helps them to be in balance. It harmonizes and soothes the body and mind, leaving you feeling calm. It's particularly good to do if you can't sleep.

1. Sit in a chair and close your eyes.

2. Place your hand on your nose, with your thumb on one nostril and your ring finger on the other.

3. Close off one nostril at a time without moving your hand!

4. Starting with closing the right nostril, breathe out through your left nostril (always start with an exhale) then inhale through the left nostril.

5. Swap nostrils by exhaling through the right nostril and inhaling through the right nostril.

Breathe normally—not too deeply. Don't worry if you need to blow your nose a lot.

Note: Always consult with a doctor if you suffer from any illness or are pregnant before doing any yoga exercises.

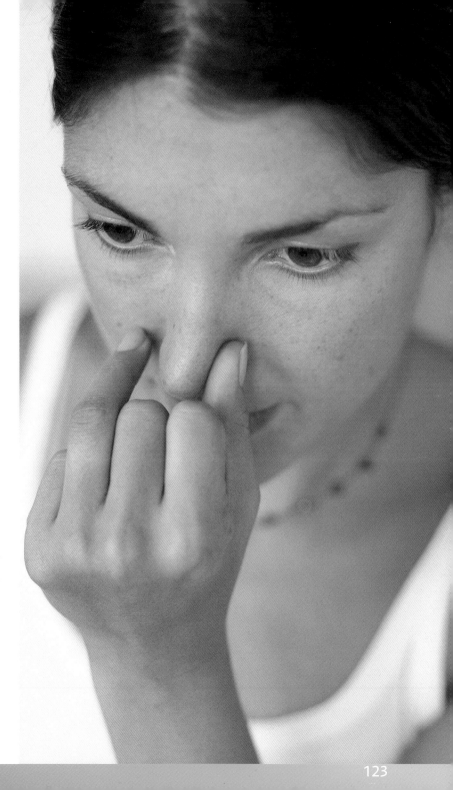

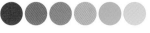

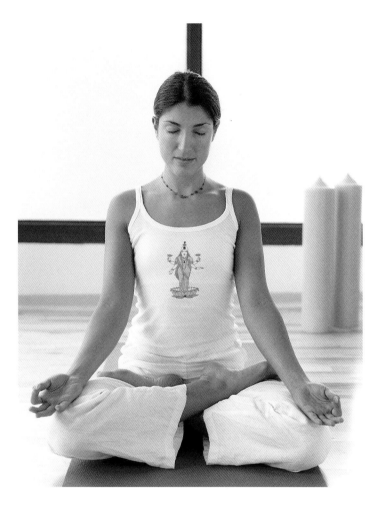

Sitting lotus

1. Sit with your legs crossed.

2. Rest your feet on the opposite calves (if you find this difficult, try the half-lotus, in which you rest just one foot on the opposite calf).

3. Put the back of your hands on your knees with your thumb and first finger touching to make an *0*.

4. Close your eyes and focus on the ground beneath you.

5. Relax your jaw and let your tongue rest on the roof of your mouth.

6. Imagine that your spine is being stretched up to the sky.

7. Breathe deeply and slowly through your nose while thinking of something positive or saying "Om."

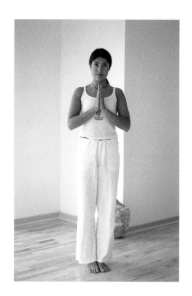

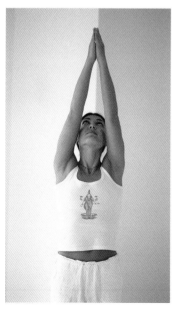

Sun salutation

This yoga position allows energy to flow throughout the whole body. It warms and invigorates the body and increases blood flow to the head. It is also a good stretching and strengthening exercise for the arms, back, legs, shoulders, and buttocks. It helps to oxygenate the body and improve circulation, relieves tension, and releases energy. It also improves flexibility and body tone. Go as far as you can with each motion without strain or pain. Start by doing it once and then gradually increase to ten times.

1. Stand with your feet together, arms by your sides, looking straight ahead. Bring your hands together in a praying position at your chest and then exhale.

2. Inhale as you bring your arms straight up over your head. With your palms still together, stretch up as high as you can and look up at your thumbs.

3. Exhale, keeping your arms straight as you bend forward, allowing your hands to reach the floor on either side of your feet, with your head relaxed down.

4. Inhale and step so you are in a lunge position with your left leg extended back. Keep your

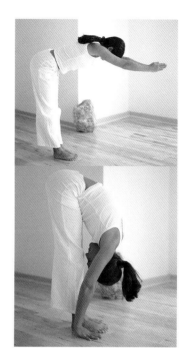

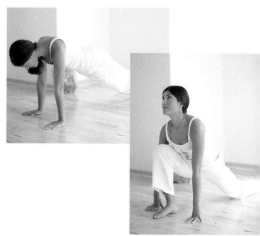

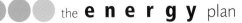

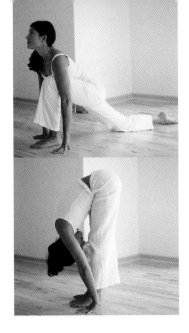

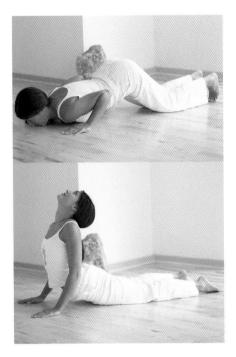

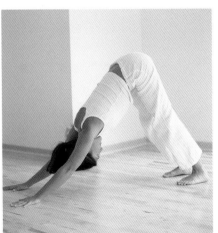

hands to either side of your right knee and keep them firmly on the floor. Look upward, stretching your back and chest. Step your right leg back.

5. Exhale, lower your knees to the floor, and then lower your chest down toward the floor with a straight back. Then inhale and straighten your arms and look up while bending back as far as you can comfortably go.

6. Exhale and push your hips up into an inverted *V*. Your arms should be shoulder-width apart and your palms facing forward. Keep your feet and heels flat on the floor.

7. Inhale and lunge forward, moving your left leg between your hands, and look upward, stretching your back. Exhale and step your right leg forward between your hands. Keep your legs together and straighten them.

8. Inhale. Come up, vertebra by vertebra, with your hands raising out to the side and then above your head, meeting in a prayer position. Look up at your hands.

9. Exhale and bring your hands to a prayer position in front of chest.

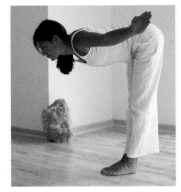

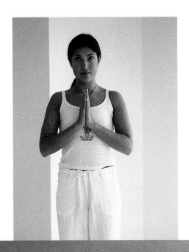

The energy triangle

This exercise opens up the hips and shoulders and allows the energy to flow smoothly. The good news is that it also helps to shape your waist and makes you more flexible.

1. Stand with your feet apart and inhale through your nose.

2. Stretch your arms out to the side, like a star.

3. Turn your left foot ninety degrees to the side and breathe out through your nose.

4. Breathe in through your nose and bend down sideways until your left hand reaches your ankle. Stretch your right hand up to the sky look up at your hand.

5. Breathe out through your nose. Come back to standing position, turn your foot back to the front, and repeat for the other side.

6. Repeat five times.

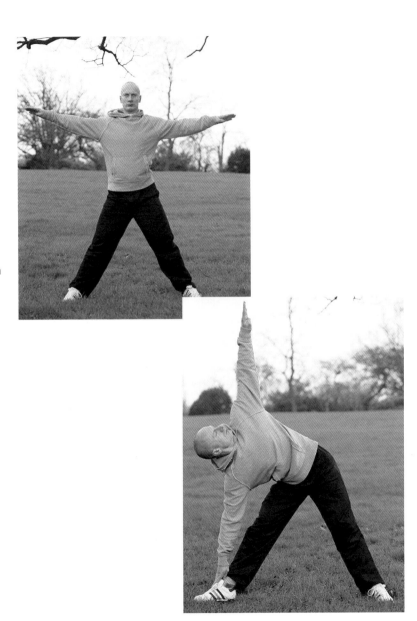

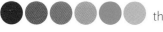
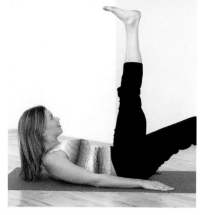

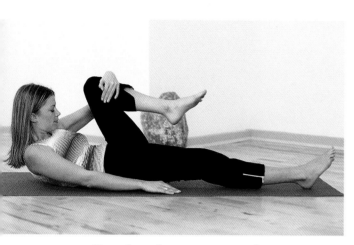

3. Inhale and gently lift your head toward your leg.

4. Exhale and lower your head. Inhale.

5. Exhale and lower your leg.

6. Repeat three times for both legs.

The half-shoulder stand (right)

This posture is very good for increasing energy, as it helps blood circulation. It also helps aching legs and low blood pressure, and elimination of waste in the bowel. The thyroid gland is also stimulated, helping to produce hormones from the endocrine system (if thyroxine is low, it can often cause low energy). Women should not do this exercise during a period. Because it is an inverted position, it gives the organs a rest.

1. Lie on your back with your arms by your side, palms down.

2. Inhale, bringing your hips and legs off the ground, supported by your hands.

3. Bring your knees to your forehead; if you are comfortable you can extend your legs first to the ceiling and then, so that your legs are at a forty-five-degree angle to your body, hold the position and breathe normally. Keep your neck straight. Do not strain. Inhale.

4. Exhale and slowly roll back to the floor.

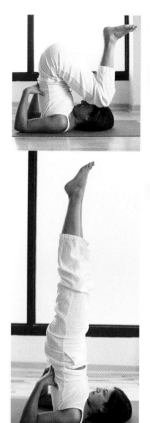

Head to knee pose (above)

Helps with constipation and irritable bowel.

1. Lie on your back with your legs straight.

2. Bend your right leg toward your chest and hug it with your right arm.

3. Breathe in and lift your head in toward your knee. Hold and breathe.

4. Exhale and lower your head. Inhale. Exhale and lower your leg.

5. Repeat three times for both legs.

Leg raises (top right)

1. Lie on the floor with your legs straight.

2. Inhale and lift your right leg with your foot flexed so that it is at right angles with your body, but do not strain. You can bend your other leg if you find this too difficult. Exhale.

The fish (below)

1. Lie on your back with your arms by your side.

2. Place your palms, facing down, under your bottom, squeeze elbows in toward each other, and keep your legs straight.

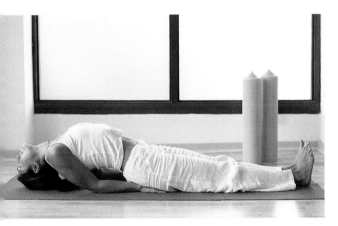

3. Inhale and put the weight of your body on your forearms and elbows. Keep your feet flexed.

4. Lift your chest (arch your back) and lower your head slowly, then rest the crown of your head on the floor so that you are looking behind you. The pressure on your head should be light and the majority of the weight held by your arms.

5. Hold for five to ten breaths, or as long as you can while breathing deeply, then exhale as you come out of the posture.

The bridge (below right)

Helps to strengthen the spine and make it more flexible.

1. Lie on the floor with your knees bent, your ankles under your knees, your feet hip-width apart, and your arms beside you.

2. Place your palms on the floor, clasping your hands under your back and pulling your shoulders downward.

3. Inhale and lift your hips as high as you can so that you are resting on your shoulders, making a bridge. You can put your hands under your waist to help lift you higher onto your shoulders. Make sure your head, neck, and feet are still flat on the floor. Use your arms and feet to support you by pushing them down into the floor. Breathe normally and hold the posture for a few seconds.

4. Exhale and slowly lower your back, vertebra by vertebra, bringing your hips down last, until you are flat on the floor.

5. Relax for a few deep breaths, then repeat twice.

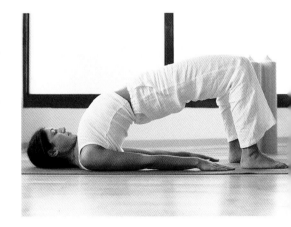

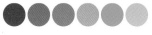
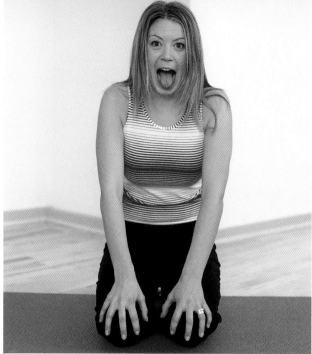

Hand clasp (below)

This posture also opens the chest, stretches the back, and helps the shoulders.

1. Kneel on the floor, sitting on your heels.

2. Put one arm behind your back and reach up

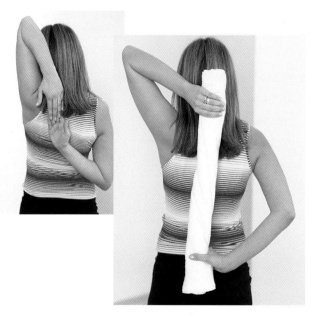

as far as you can toward your shoulders with your arm bent and your palm facing out. Bring your other arm over its shoulder so that the hands meet. Try to hold hands, but if you can't reach, use a towel and hold it between your hands.

3. Pull up and down; hold for a few seconds.

4. Repeat for the other side.

The lion (above)

This pose stimulates the blood and energy to the face, helping you not only to feel more energized, but to look more energetic, as well. It's also good if you are coming down with a cold.

1. Kneel on the floor, sitting on your heels.

2. Put the back of your hands on your knees, spreading your fingers. Inhale through your nose.

3. Leaning slightly forward, exhale through your mouth and make a "Haa" sound while sticking your tongue out as far as it will go.

4. Stretch out your fingers and look up at the space between your eyes. Hold for a few seconds and then close your mouth.

Don't worry if you feel a bit silly doing this pose!

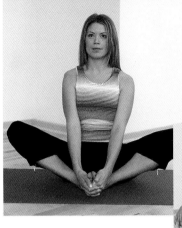

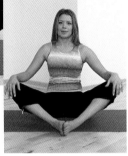

The butterfly (above)

1. Sit upright, keeping the soles of your feet together.

2. Hold on to your feet with your hands. Slowly and gently bounce your knees up and down, going as close to the floor as possible.

3. After a few minutes, put your hands on your knees and gently push them toward the floor.

Forward stretch (below)

This helps your nervous system and solar plexus.

1. Sit on the floor with your legs together, stretched out in front of you.

2. Sit upright with your feet flexed.

3. Inhale and lift your arms up over your head and look up at your hands.

4. Exhale, lengthen the spine, and bend forward from the hips, moving your chest toward your legs. Only go as far as you can. Try to keep your back straight and lengthened. Hold for a few seconds.

5. Inhale and slowly come back up.

Backward stretch (right)

This is great for increasing your energy and good to do after the forward stretch.

1. Lie on your front.

2. Lift your weight up onto your forearms, with your elbows under your shoulders.

3. Pull your shoulders back.

4. Look straight ahead and hold for a few seconds. Don't forget to breathe.

5. Exhaling, lower yourself down and rest.

6. Repeat twice more.

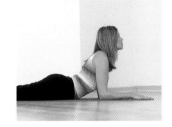

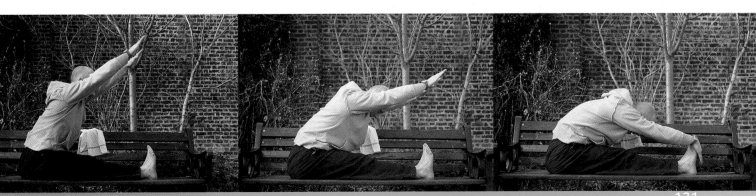

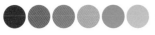
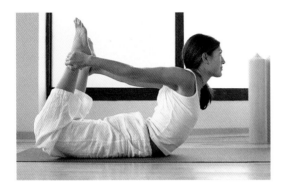

The bow (above)

This is great for increasing energy and gives the internal organs a massage.

1. Lie on your front and bring your feet back toward your bottom, knees hip-width apart.

2. Reach back with your hands to hold your ankles. Exhale.

3. Inhale and lift your chest and head and pull your shoulders back while still holding your ankles. Also lift your knees, thighs, and hips so that you are resting on your abdomen. Use your legs to pull yourself up.

4. Arch your back and look upward, or straight ahead if it hurts your neck.

5. Take three deep breaths (you might rock slightly as you do so).

6. Exhale and come slowly down and relax into the pose of a child (below).

The pose of a child (below)

As your head is below your heart in this pose, it circulates blood to the brain and gives you energy.

1. Kneel down with your bottom resting on your heels.

2. Bend forward and rest your forehead on the floor.

3. Put your arms at your sides with your palms by your feet, facing upward.

4. Breathe deeply and relax.

NOTE: those who suffer from high blood pressure should not do this exercise without seeking medical advice.

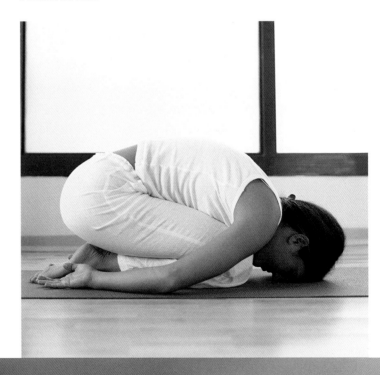

Energy boosts during the day when at work

Sitting at a desk all day, particularly at a computer, will make your shoulders, neck, and spine tense, and as a result you will feel achy and tired. The lack of movement in a stuffy office also slows down the flow of blood and qi around your body. This is when most people reach for a caffeine pick-me-up or a sweet snack.

It is all too easy to get sucked into your work, to almost become your work and forget about taking care of your body. Most of us live in our heads rather than our bodies and have no idea even how our bodies are feeling until maybe at the end of the day when we finally stop and realize how hungry, thirsty, tired, stiff, and achy we feel.

Try and stop just for a minute every hour to touch base with your body. How are you feeling? Is your neck tense? Are you clenching your jaw? Are you hungry or thirsty? Do you need water or a good, nourishing meal instead of a greasy sandwich? Does your back or bottom ache from sitting too long? Do you need a stretch, are you tired? Do your eyes need a rest?

It's not always possible to give in to every need of the body, but try to give yourself some of the quick fixes that are good for you, like a glass of water, some fruit, stretching, rolling your neck, or taking a break for a few minutes. You will find that it is easier to work and concentrate if you are relaxed and happy.

● Try taking regular breaks. Walk around the office to get a glass of water or go to the bathroom. Try walking just out to the front door (or at least to a window), take some deep breaths, and then walk back to your desk.

● You can also get in a twenty-minute walk every day by walking to work or getting off the train or bus early or parking your car farther away and walking the rest of the way.

● When you go to the bathroom (or in the office if you can), do the standing yoga stretch (page 134). It can also be done outside. It helps to relax the shoulders, neck, and spine, and it allows the vertebrae to stretch instead of being pushed on top of each other. This, in turn, allows the spinal fluid to flow smoothly and nourishes the spinal cord and brain, thus helping with concentration and also lifting your spirits.

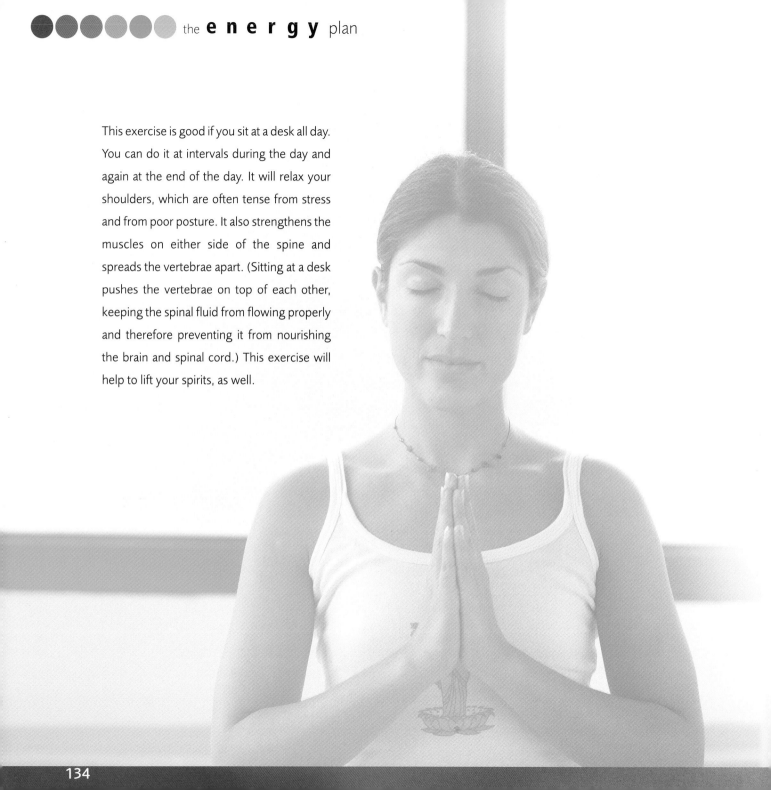

This exercise is good if you sit at a desk all day. You can do it at intervals during the day and again at the end of the day. It will relax your shoulders, which are often tense from stress and from poor posture. It also strengthens the muscles on either side of the spine and spreads the vertebrae apart. (Sitting at a desk pushes the vertebrae on top of each other, keeping the spinal fluid from flowing properly and therefore preventing it from nourishing the brain and spinal cord.) This exercise will help to lift your spirits, as well.

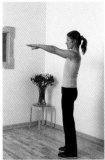

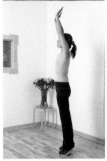

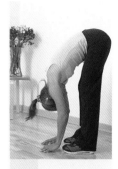

STANDING YOGA STRETCH AT DESK

1. Stand with your feet hip-width apart and your knees slightly bent and shoulders relaxed.

2. Inhale through your nose and lift your arms up straight in front of your body to shoulder height.

3. Stretch your arms up to above your head, with your palms facing the sky; imagine that you are pushing the sky away. Go up onto your toes.

4. Slowly lower yourself down off your toes and firmly ground your feet.

5. Breathe out through your nose and bend down and touch the floor or your toes. Let your body be as loose as possible.

6. Breathe in through your nose and straighten up, one vertebra at a time, until you are back in the starting position.

7. Repeat five to ten times.

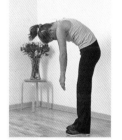

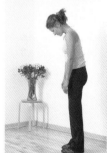

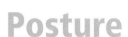

Posture

Our posture can affect how we feel emotionally and physically, and therefore has an effect on our energy.

Posture is a very powerful thing. If you change your posture, you can change your mood, and you can tell a lot about a person and how they are feeling by the way they hold themselves. The more strained or nervous you feel, the more you tend to close up your body, for example by folding your arms or crossing your legs. This cuts the energy flow and the longer you stay locked in that position, the more nervous you will feel. Conversely, by opening up your posture you restore energy flow and as a consequence you will feel more relaxed.

The Alexander Technique is based on the close connection between posture and mood, and between your posture and your physical health. When you are tired you are more likely to slump in a chair, and this will make you feel more tired

because you restrict many organs in the body. Your heart has to work harder and it will become harder to breathe due to the tension that you feel around your ribs.

When we are stressed we often have hunched shoulders, and this hampers our breathing, creating muscle tension. In the long term, this can make the diaphragm too stiff and tense, and hard to expand or stretch when you try to relax and breathe properly.

If you sit in a slouched position, your spine is sloped backward and your shoulders and the top of your back are under stress to try and keep your head up. The tension and lactic acid buildup causes a sore neck and shoulders. If you sat in the proper position, your head would balance naturally on your shoulders, resulting in no tension and allowing your rib cage to expand easily when you breathe.

Similarly, if you slump at your desk at work all day with rounded shoulders, you will have neck pain as again your neck muscles are being overworked to keep the head erect. You are also shortening and tightening the muscles across the chest, preventing proper breathing.

However, if you sit with a strong back and

stomach and relaxed shoulders, your body will be able to cope better and you will feel less tense and tired at the end of the day.

If you have had a poor posture for many years, then the correct postures will feel very strange at first. Try to think about your posture throughout the day and correct it whenever you remember to. Soon, using the correct posture will become second nature.

Standing

- Stand with pelvis centred correctly.
- Use your stomach muscles to keep equilibrium.
- Keep your knees relaxed, not locked.
- Straighten your shoulders; they should be held down and relaxed (shrug them a few times to loosen them).
- Neck and head should sit comfortably on your spine; don't lean your head forward or down.

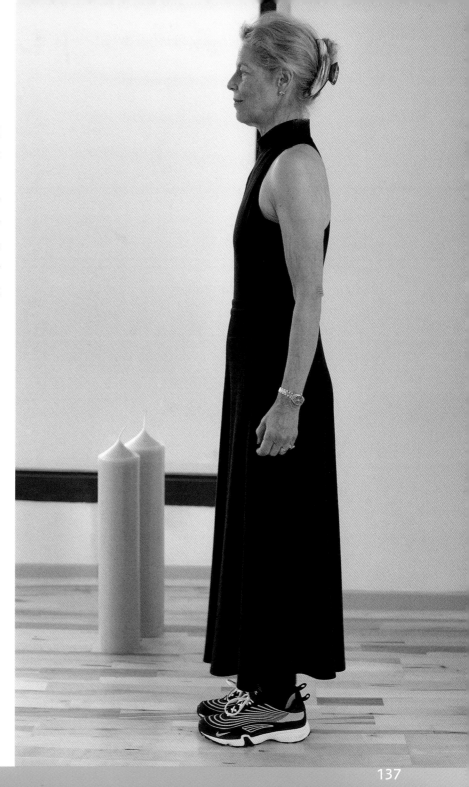

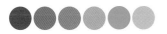

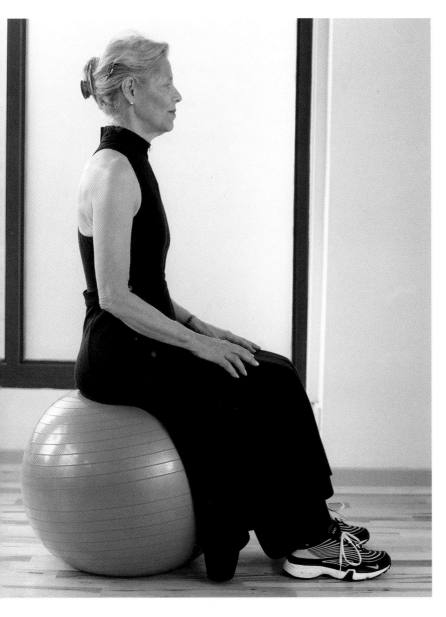

Sitting

● Try to get a chair with good support for the lower back.

● Sit with your tailbone at the back of the chair.

● Your feet should be flat on the floor; mid- and lower back need to be kept strong to avoid slumping.

● Shoulders should be relaxed and down.

● Head and neck should sit loosely.

● Work should be at a correct height and distance away so you can keep this position.

● Take short rests every hour, walk around the room, get some fresh air, or at least do some stretching exercises while sitting.

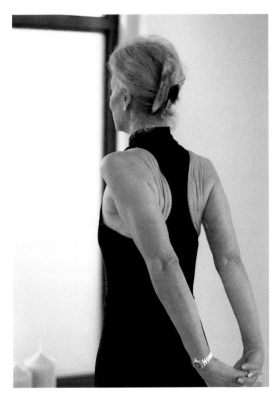

Chest stretch (above)

This is good if your breathing is tight or if your shoulders tend to be hunched.

1. Stand with your hands clasped behind your back, palms facing upward.

2. Shoulders should be down and relaxed.

3. Bring your hands out, away from your back, so that you feel the stretch across your chest and shoulders.

Spinal stretch (below)

This is very good if you are very stiff.

1. Sit on a chair.

2. Breathe out and drop your head and neck down toward your chest until you feel a stretch along your spine.

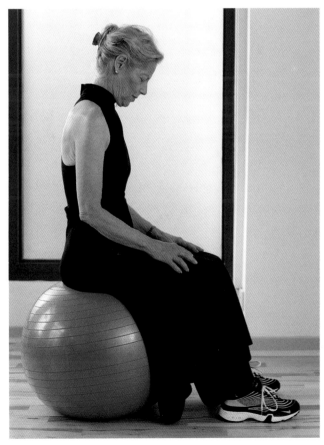

Exercise according to Ayurveda

Some traditions, like Ayurveda, believe that different types of people should exercise differently.

Vata

Vata people tend to be slim, with an active mind. They are often restless and talk a lot. Everything they do, they do quickly—walking, eating, talking, etc. They find it difficult to sit still, and they sleep very lightly. They learn quickly, but also forget quickly, and have a vivid imagination. They are very creative and sensitive.

Exercise for vata people

Sports that involve sprinting, running, and quick movements. All sports suit vata types, especially ones that require speed and agility.

Pitta

Pitta people usually have an average appetite and build, and they walk and talk at average speed. They are natural leaders, strong-minded, fiery, and quick-tempered. They have good coordination and are very competitive.

Exercise for pitta people

Competitive sports suit them best, so pitta people should try team or league sports, or exercise with a partner.

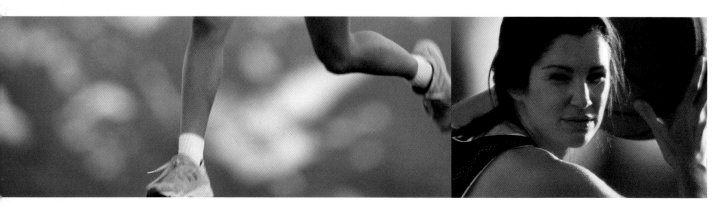

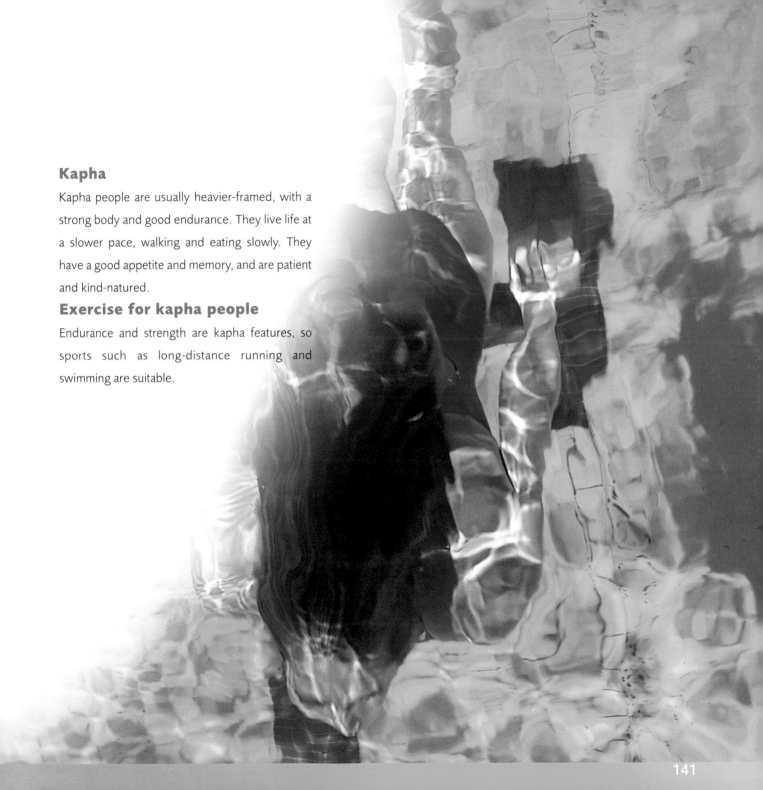

Kapha

Kapha people are usually heavier-framed, with a strong body and good endurance. They live life at a slower pace, walking and eating slowly. They have a good appetite and memory, and are patient and kind-natured.

Exercise for kapha people

Endurance and strength are kapha features, so sports such as long-distance running and swimming are suitable.

Vibrational energy

Many New Age philosophies believe that even if your diet is good and you exercise regularly, you may still have no energy. This may happen if the energy either around you or in your home or workplace is not right in some way. They seek to address the nonphysical, or spiritual, dimension of energy, and I have included some of them in this book to provide the most rounded and holistic approach possible to improving your energy levels.

Crystals

For thousands of years, crystals have been used for their powers. Buddhist monks carved crystal balls out of quartz and claimed they were the gem of enlightenment. Today people use crystals for their healing qualities. They may be held, worn, or placed strategically around the home or office.

People who work with crystals say that if you work or live around a lot of electrical equipment, you will start to feel irritable, low, and fatigued, and will possibly suffer from increasing health complaints. They say that placing quartz crystals around and on items such as computers or

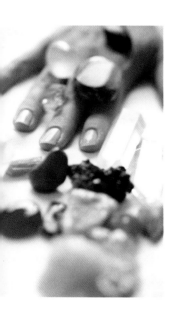

televisions helps to absorb some of the negative energy that they emit.

Crystals are believed to store energy from their place of origin, and many have been known to have properties to help alleviate ailments such as fatigue, depression, and stress. If they are kept clean and programmed, they can be very invigorating, whether they are used somewhere in the home or during a treatment from an experienced healer. Crystals are believed to give off positive healing energies that can rebalance our bodies as they match the energy of the human aura.

Crystals generate, store, and give off electromagnetic energy. Each one has its own particular energy that has a specific healing effect on mind, body, and spirit. Quartz, for example, is known to generate small amounts of piezoelectricity, which is used to power computers, and in healing terms it is used to help you think more clearly and speed up healing. Amber has a more calming property and helps with depression, moonstone helps to balance hormones and emotions, ruby helps build the blood, and tiger's-eye can be useful for overcoming fatigue.

THE COLORS OF AN AURA

These are basic guidelines:

Purple/violet: spiritual, religious, idealistic

Indigo: inspiration, wisdom, sensitive, spiritual

Blue: intellectual, intelligent, rational and logical thinker, intuitive

Turquoise: dynamic, energetic, good organizer, communicative, likes to influence others

Green: calm, balanced, kind, caring, gentle (dark green = deceit or jealousy)

Yellow: fun, loving, cheerful, full of vitality, compassionate, optimistic

Orange: full of vitality, warm, generous, someone who has power, inspirational

Gold: well balanced, kind, generous, great spiritual leader

Red: physical, full of vitality, ambitious, sensual, high sex drive

Pink: true romantic, modest, shy, gentle

Brown: unsettled, materialistic, negative or just in a bad mood

Gray: depressed, afraid, full of morbid thoughts, low energy

Black: has deep-rooted problems, unpleasant character

White: illness or drug abuse

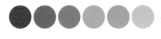

If you think you might like to wear a crystal, quartz is a good choice since it will help keep your mind clear. However, if you find that you are particularly drawn to another type of crystal, you will probably find that it is an important and relevant one to you.

The aura

The aura is a subtle energy that vibrates around everyone's body. Understanding auras is a key to understanding why, for example, just being around someone with an overpowering aura or personality can leave you feeling depleted and lacking in energy.

Seeing and sensing auras gives you a unique insight into how people are feeling both physically and emotionally, and interacting with others becomes much more efficient and productive. The aura cannot lie. If you feel uncomfortable around someone, your aura will shrink away from them. If someone is aggressive or overpowering, their aura can take over yours. If you are happy with someone, your auras will meet or even merge into one.

Seeing auras

Start by looking at the aura of a healthy tree. Look up at a tree, preferably on a clear day, and let your eyes drift slightly out of focus. You will begin to notice a faint shimmer around the tree. Practice doing the same thing with plants against a white wall. First look at a healthy plant and compare it with one that is dying. Look at animals, too, and then start practicing on friends, preferably against a white wall. You can also practice anytime, anywhere—while in a line, at work, on a train, in class. You can also assess your own aura by looking at yourself in a mirror.

Once you get used to seeing the aura, you will notice different colors in it. If the color is bright and clear, it usually means the person is healthy and happy. Dirty dark colors tend to mean physical illness, tiredness, or an emotional problem. A flash of color can indicate an emotion that is out of control.

Chakras

Understanding your chakras will help you understand your own energy. Chakras are monitors of our physical and mental well-being, and each one relates to a particular area of the body. Your chakras spin at different frequencies. If each chakra spins at the correct frequency, you will feel centered, balanced, and energized, and will radiate perfect health. Blocks in energy, however, will prevent a chakra from vibrating as it should, and ill health and fatigue will result. These blocks can be cleared by visualizations, healing, and exercises such as yoga, which, in turn, will allow you to feel more energized physically, emotionally, and spiritually.

In Sanskrit, chakra means "wheel" or "vortex." It is a spinning wheel that takes in energy and feeds all the other areas of the physical and subtle body on a physical, emotional, and spiritual level. There are seven major chakras, each of which has its own location and emotions, organs, colors, sound, and level of consciousness associated with it. The seven chakras run in a line up the middle of the body and head, and send energy along channels known as nadis. There are 72,000 nadis in the body.

The chakras emanate energy away from the body, forming the aura, which can be seen by some people as a colored light that surrounds the body. Many healers work with their patients' chakras and aura, and are able to see how a person is feeling both physically and emotionally by looking at the colors and vibrations of their electrical field of energy (the aura).

Your lower chakras relate to your more earthbound emotional states and the higher ones to your spiritual states. Your chakras are always either open or blocked; when a person dies, their chakras are closed. A blocked chakra takes in less prana (energy), resulting, as we know, in poor health and fatigue. If a chakra is too open, it will take in more energy than you are able to cope with, making you feel overwhelmed.

The seven chakras:

1. Muladhara: the root/base chakra
2. Swadhishthana: the navel/sacral chakra
3. Manipura: the solar plexus chakra
4. Anahata: the heart chakra
5. Vishuddha: the throat chakra
6. Ajna: the third-eye chakra
7. Sahasrara: the crown chakra

1 The root/base chakra

COLOR: RED

Emotion: anchor and foundation, grounded in the present, having the will to live

Physical: adrenal system, lower bowels

Element : earth vibrates to a solid frequency

Location: base of spine

Blocked: lacking energy, weak constitution, feeling depersonalized, fear of letting go, daydreaming

Too open: very materialistic, not spiritual

Balanced: accepting yourself, secure, healthy, lots of energy and enthusiasm

Healing: to balance this chakra, try visualizing; for example, breathing in red light, filling your body with red light, etc. Meditation is not as good for this chakra, but is better for balancing the upper chakras. It is vital to have your root chakra balanced (like the roots of a tree). Any activity that puts you in contact with the earth or helps you feel rooted in the present is good. Try walking (especially barefoot), gardening, dancing, and pottery, or wearing red clothes below the waist.

2 The navel/sacral chakra

COLOR: ORANGE

Emotion: creation of life, sensual energy, and sexual relations

Physical: reproductive system: ovaries, uterus, testicles and prostrate, vaginal and pelvic infections, PMS, male infertility, endometriosis, fatigue

Element: water

Location: between the lower abdomen and navel

Blocked: a disruption in your sexual relationships

Too open: envy, lust, fear, confusion, overdependence on partner

Balanced: a balance between the male and female energies (ha and tha, or yin and yang), independent and whole, good sexual relationships

Healing: trust and enjoy all your senses; visualizations with all the senses, for example, smelling something nice, seeing something energizing, feeling something, hearing water, etc. Breathe in orange light. Pelvic tilts are good, as is wearing orange from the waist down.

3 The solar plexus chakra

COLOR: YELLOW

Emotion: center for your major emotions, wants, desires, ego, and ambitions; this is where your sense of "I am" comes from

Physical: pancreas, stomach, gallbladder, spleen, and small intestine; digestive disorders and eating disorders; hypoglycemia; chronic fatigue; diabetes; pancreatic problems; indigestion and irritable bowel. Your solar plexus is your true energy center, since you get your stamina from digesting food. This is why the right food is very important for helping you beat fatigue.

Element: fire

Location: around the solar plexus

Blocked: selfish and unfeeling, lack of willpower and drive, depressed, exhausted, and stressed

Too open: overemotional, greedy, angry, aggressive, always looking after other people's feelings instead of your own, oversubmissive, passive, powerless, which can lead to resentment and exhaustion

Balanced: feeling centered, flexible, happy, warm, confident, good sense of humor, spontaneous, playful, able to express emotions

Healing: you need to learn to separate your own emotions and responsibilities from other people's. Must not block your feelings and be open to new experiences and adventures, take risks, ground yourself. Do stress management techniques such as yoga and meditation. Visualize a mirror between you and anyone who you think might drain you of energy; for example, if they are very depressed and complaining to you, or very angry. Breathe gold sunlight into your solar plexus and then spread it around the rest of your body.

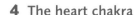 the **e n e r g y** plan

4 The heart chakra

COLOR: GREEN

Emotion: joy and sadness, love, harmony and compassion, intimacy

Physical: blood and circulation, heart, lungs, breasts, thymus

Element: air

Location: in the heart/chest

Blocked: difficulty in keeping up a loving relationship, detached, cold, reserved, short of breath, heart problems, immune system problems, asthma

Too open: too sensitive, worrying about other people's needs until you become exhausted

Balanced: compassionate, loving, empathetic, peaceful, balanced

Healing: any exercise that helps open the chest area. Surround yourself with nature and physical touch from loved ones. Visualize the color green pouring into the heart chakra and then emanating around the rest of your body.

5 The throat chakra

COLOR: BLUE

Emotion: how you communicate and express yourself to the outside world

Physical: thyroid gland, throat and voice, ears, neck, tightness of the jaw, endocrine system

Location: in the throat

Blocked: problems with words, speaking quietly, sarcastic, cynical, hostile, tired from not speaking your mind and trying to be someone that you are not, asthma, hyperventilation, bronchitis, hypothyroidism, throat problems, mouth ulcers, hearing problems

Too open: talkative, dominating conversations without saying anything of value

Balanced: interacting with the world through communication, talking, listening, and reading, expressing your true feelings clearly

Healing: need to use your voice—singing, chanting, humming, or shouting; sound therapy and voice work; meditation; massage

6 The third-eye chakra

COLOR: INDIGO BLUE

Emotion: imagination and concentration, spirituality

Physical: eyes, brain and nervous system, pineal and pituitary glands, hypothalamus

Location: in the forehead, between the eyebrows

Blocked: tiredness and mental fatigue, headaches, learning difficulties, negative thinking, poor concentration, confusion, delusions, psychosis

Too open: anxiety, clairvoyant

Balanced: creative, intuitive, good at visualizing

Healing: painting and drawing, writing down dreams, meditation, breathing through alternating nostrils

7 The crown chakra

COLOR: VIOLET AND WHITE

Emotion: open-minded, thoughtful and wise, analyzing and assimilating information, cynical, greedy and materialistic, intellectual, living in your head, losing touch with body

Physical: upper brain, pituitary and pineal glands

Location: in the cerebral cortex of the brain

Blocked: depression; difficulty accepting life; trapped in your body; no spiritual connection or direction, making you feel drained and exhausted

Too open: too spiritual and unable to relate to the real world, anxiety and fear

Balanced: acceptance and peace

Healing: meditation, open to new ideas and information, look into spirituality/religion, physical exercise, massage, gardening

The chakras in the lower half of the body create energy for the physical body and sensations to go with it, whereas those located in the upper half are associated with spiritual and emotional energy.

The chakra balance

1. Stand with your feet hip-width apart and imagine a rope from the center of the top of your head up to the sky keeping you upright.

2. Make sure your body is relaxed; close your eyes and concentrate on your breathing.

3. Imagine that above your head there is a shimmering ball of violet energy and that you are breathing into it.

4. Imagine that you are breathing in from the violet ball of energy, and when you breathe out, the energy moves through your body down to your feet, where it exits into the earth.

5. Repeat five times.

6. Imagine another ball of dark red energy pulsating at a steady beat. Breathe into this red ball of energy, and as you breathe in, take the red energy up your feet and through the base of your spine, up to the top of your head.

7. Repeat five times.

8. Stand still for a minute; allow your breathing to come back to normal. Slowly open your eyes.

A shamanic visualization for increasing energy

1. Close your eyes and concentrate on your breathing.

2. Imagine that a huge and powerful eagle is in front of you looking at you with his all-seeing eye. Nod and thank him.

3. The eagle turns and spreads his wings, allowing you to use his sharp, far-sighted vision.

4. Now imagine a huge bear behind you. Turn and look into her eyes and notice her strength and weight and claws; she is very protective and will protect your back. Thank her for her powerful presence behind you.

5. To your right a coyote is sniffing, his tongue hanging out as if he were laughing. He is smart and quick and good at negotiating. He can help in any difficult situation, but don't let him become too clever for his own good.

6. On your left you see a buffalo, solid and dependable, which makes you feel grounded and stable.

7. Say "thank you" to your guardians, and if you want to follow tradition, you can offer them a pinch of tobacco or cornmeal.

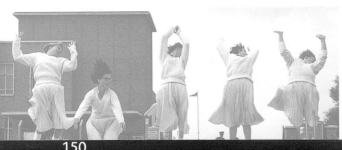

Energy in relationships

Just as we need the energy to flow smoothly in our homes and bodies, we also need it to flow smoothly in our relationships with other people. Relationships are a vital part of our lives and can be a huge source of energy.

Communication and interaction with other people can be exhilarating, stimulating, and energizing. Sex is energizing, and it has been found that people who have regular sex lives live longer, and are happier and healthier than those who don't. However, relationships can also cause a lot of stress, especially those with a partner, since they bring emotions such as jealousy, suspicion, mistrust, resentment, misunderstanding, anger, sadness, fear, depression, and guilt. Small amounts of stress that can later be resolved through an argument is normal, but constant stress is draining, depressing, and robs you of your energy.

Different people have different effects on your energy levels. Some seem to zap and drain your energy, while others boost it. Obviously you want to surround yourself as far as is possible with people who boost your energy, encourage you, and are positive toward you and your life.

Sometimes, though, a relationship with a friend or family member or partner may still be very important to you, even though they drain you of all your energy.

In such cases, it is important to acknowledge that the person has this effect on you so that you can protect yourself and perhaps not see them on days when you feel particularly exhausted. When you do see them, try to imagine that you are in a protective bubble that they cannot get through, or imagine a mirror between the two of you that reflects their energy back at them.

If someone makes you very angry, instead of holding on to the anger, which will later create a block in your energy, try some of these techniques to let the anger out:

- Go for a walk and, making sure that no one is around, shout at the top of your voice.
- Get a pillow and punch it with all the anger you feel instead of bottling it up.
- Write down what you feel either in a diary or a letter that you will never send to someone who has made you very angry.
- Stamp your feet repeatedly while making a loud noise until you feel better.

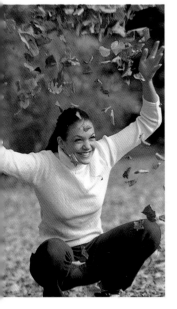

Express yourself

Body workers have found that repressed emotions are stored in different parts of the body. For example, problems with your throat, jaw, and mouth are due to not being able to say what you feel or not being heard. If we hold on to all the emotions from our past and present, it is hard for our energy to circulate and be at its optimum level. Expressing your feelings is very important in terms of how much energy you have. Next time you see someone who is angry or upset, imagine how much energy it must take to hide their emotions, or to keep pushing them down pretending that everything is fine. Pretending to be somebody that you are not is exhausting.

Keeping energy in a relationship

○ Try to be with people who tend to energize and encourage you.

○ Keep your sense of self and self-esteem (don't let others take over, dominate, and engulf you; make sure you live your own life and make your own decisions).

○ Keep communicating. If you don't keep talking things through that are bothering you in a relationship, they can feel and get bigger, causing you to worry and zapping your energy.

○ Don't take each other for granted; try to remember what it was that you first saw in your partner that attracted you to him/her.

○ If things seem to have been wrong between you and your partner for a long time and you are finding it hard to resolve the problems, go to a relationship counselor together.

Happiness

Happiness means different things for different people, but there is one thing that is true of everyone: When you experience what you feel is happiness, you are energized. If you are not happy with your life, you will not function well. Negative emotions can reduce energy and positive emotions increase it. By making yourself feel happy, you can help to build your energy.

You can practice being happy by reacting to your day in a positive and cheerful way. Think of things that made you happy today and schedule them into your day tomorrow. Don't wait for happiness to come to you—engineer it. If you can't pinpoint what makes you happy, try keeping a mood diary and write down things that made you happy; for example, spending time with a friend, watching a good movie, painting, or buying something for yourself.

Here are a few tips to keep you feeling happy:

● Remember to count your blessings regularly and to think of the positive aspects of your life.

● Compare yourself to people who are less fortunate than you.

● Spend time with people who make you feel good/happy.

● Appreciate your surroundings.

● Learn to recognize moments of happiness, however brief.

● Don't indulge in self-pity.

● Always try to keep a positive frame of mind.

● Try not to blame your problems on others.

● Exercise regularly. Exercise releases endorphins in your brain, which makes you feel happy.

● Find at least one thing each day that will make you feel happy.

Feng shui

Feng shui is the ancient Chinese art and science of placement, and its main concept is energy flow—feng shui is to your home and surroundings what acupuncture is to your body. If the energy flow in your home is smooth and harmonious, you will reap the benefits. If your home is very cluttered, the flow of energy will be upset. Where there is a mess, the energy becomes stuck, eventually

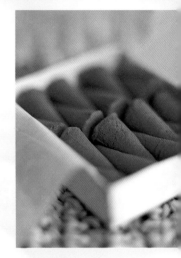

leaving a pile of stagnant energy. Not only will it make you feel tired and possibly unwell, you will also find that things will become "stuck" in your life and you might end up feeling very frustrated. Below is a simple feng shui map. Place it over a map of your house to work out the location of each corresponding area.

Then start packing. Remove, give away, sell, or throw away anything that has not been worn or used in the past year. Hoarding keeps new things from coming in; you need to make space so that new energy and new things in life can enter. Then clean your home, open all the doors and windows, and allow fresh air to circulate once again. Burn sage or other essential oils to give the house a new smell and atmosphere.

Money	Success	Relationships
Elders	Unity	Creativity
Knowledge	Career	Helpful Friends

← **DOOR** →

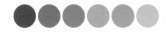

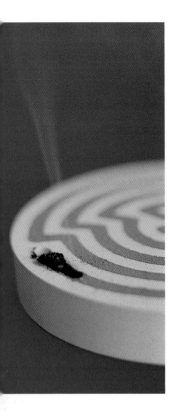

Your home should be your sanctuary, giving you the strength and stability to go out and face the world. Natural light is essential for health and energy. Basement apartments and homes on low ground surrounded by hills or tall trees deplete energy and can make you feel depressed, since there is not enough light. We need to take energy into account when decorating, choosing lighting, and positioning beds and furniture. Sharp corners, for example, and angular lines can make us feel restless. Even the position of the building itself can be significant. In China buildings are placed according to precise energetic rules.

You don't need to be a feng shui practitioner to know if a house or room feels good to live in. The atmosphere in a house soaks up the energy of the people in it, so if a couple have been arguing, angry, and unhappy in a house, their negative energy is left behind like trash. Equally, we have all been to places where it's hard to leave because the atmosphere feels so calming and safe.

Feng shui in the workplace

○ Never have your back to the door when you are sitting down—always have your desk either facing the door or preferably diagonally opposite the door. This gives you the best energy for control, authority, and concentration. If you can't change the position that your desk is in and your back has to face the door, then put up a mirror so you can see people coming into the room.

CLEARING SPACE

Many ancient cultures have traditions of clearing space in order to move energy around houses. The Chinese have the feng shui system, the Indian culture has vastu shastra, the Native American culture has the smudge ceremony, and the Balinese have bell-ringing and flower-offering ceremonies. All of these can be used to shift energy in your home. Even in the West we have space-clearing techniques: ringing church bells on wedding days or on Sundays, clearing the air with the sound; burning incense in church or homes to cleanse the air; spring cleaning after the winter (a time of hoarding) has ended.

○ Plants help keep the energy clean, and they can also take away the radiation effects of your computer. Make sure you tend to them, though.

○ Always try to have fresh flowers on your desk, because they stimulate mental activity in addition to cleaning the atmosphere.

○ It is good to have a small candle or night-light burning while you work. It helps focus the mind and brings the energy of fire into the room to help enliven your own energy.

○ Try burning rosemary oil for concentration, bergamot to uplift you, and citrus oil. You could use lavender if you are feeling very stressed.

○ A clear quartz crystal on your desk will help you feel more focused and energized, and can help remove the radiation effects of your computer.

○ Your attitude affects the energy of the work you do. If you are negative and bored with your work, that is what it will give back to you, whereas if you are stimulated and energized by it, you will leave work at the end of each day feeling great.

Simple remedies to help move energy

○ Use an ionizer or a salt crystal to take away the positive ions that can make you feel tired and irritable. A bowl of fresh water does the same, but change it regularly or it will become stagnant.

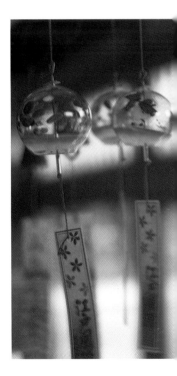

CLEARING RITUALS

○ Clapping: Clap around each corner of the room, starting at the floor and going up as high as you can. The sound might sound dull at first, but then it should become clearer. Energy gets stuck in corners and alcoves.

○ Smudging: You can buy smudge sticks (usually sage, cedar, or sweetgrass) or make your own. Light the smudge stick and blow it out so that it is smoking. You can clean your aura or other people's by blowing smoke around them. Then smudge the corners of rooms. Incense can also clean energy, though smudging is more powerful.

○ Bells and drums: Using sound for cleansing is very common. Go around your house using an instrument to make a noise, or you can use your voice.

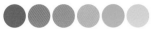

○ Use oils to help lift the energy of the house: peppermint, lemon, lemongrass, or lavender for relaxing; geranium for lifting the spirits.

○ Wind chimes help to move energy.

○ Pets and flowers add a living energy to the house, but always remember to throw away dead flowers. Spider plants positioned near a computer can help soak up the radiation and ionize the air.

○ A well-lit home helps reflect energy around the room and light up dark corners that would otherwise create a space where energy can become stuck.

○ Mirrors also reflect energy where it is missing; for example, in a room where a corner is cut off.

Colors in the home

You can change the energy in your home by changing the colors of your walls—even splashes of color help energize certain areas of the house. Some people suggest that if you have two floors or more, the lower floors should be decorated in reds, oranges, and yellows. Blues are good for bedrooms and bathrooms, and violets and indigos for bedrooms, especially on the top floor.

Red is very good for increasing the energy, but don't overdo it, as it can be overpowering.

A few red pillows and a red throw can help bring more passion into a relationship. Orange brings joy, confidence, and sociability (good for rooms used for entertaining). Yellow lifts the spirits and helps to raise the energy, which is good for rooms in the house like the kitchen, hall, living rooms, and bathrooms, and for rooms where you need to work, since it stimulates the left side of the brain. Green helps to balance and

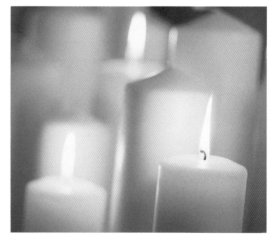

is soothing and calming (making it a good color for troubled teenagers). Blue is relaxing and peaceful, promotes rest, and helps encourage good communication, so it is a good color to use in an office at home. In the bedroom, blue can be used to help promote a good night's rest.

Balance the elements in your home

● FIRE (red and other vibrant colors)

A real fire brings vibrant energy into the house as well as warmth, strength, and peace. If you do not have a fireplace, you can use candles or crystals, hung in the windows to reflect the sunlight into your home, and you can hang mirrors so that they reflect the light already inside your home.

● EARTH (brown, terra-cotta, and brick)

Earth is grounding and strengthening. It helps us feel stable and certain of our direction in life. Salt is often put around a room or even your bed to help connect you to the earth. Crystals can also help.

● WATER (sea colors and riverbeds, very artistic with lots of paintings and clutter)

Water is purifying, cleansing, and helps rejuvenate. It is good for clearing a room of negative energies and emotions. A nice indoor waterfall can help keep the energy of the house clean; a spring-water mist spray is also good if you want to clear the energy after an argument.

● AIR (clean, airy, spacious, minimalist, and cool)

Air transforms energy; to enliven a room you can burn incense. Open the windows and allow fresh air in, even if only for a few minutes. Fans circulate air. Open space gives a feeling of airiness; it makes you feel free and full of infinite possibilities.

ENERGY CHECKLIST

To beat fatigue, try to:

● tune in to how you feel every day

● practice yoga postures regularly

● exercise regularly

● make sure you get some time to rest and relax, as well as time for yourself

● check your posture regularly

● eat well and drink lots of water

● breathe well

● meditate for twenty minutes each day

● think positively

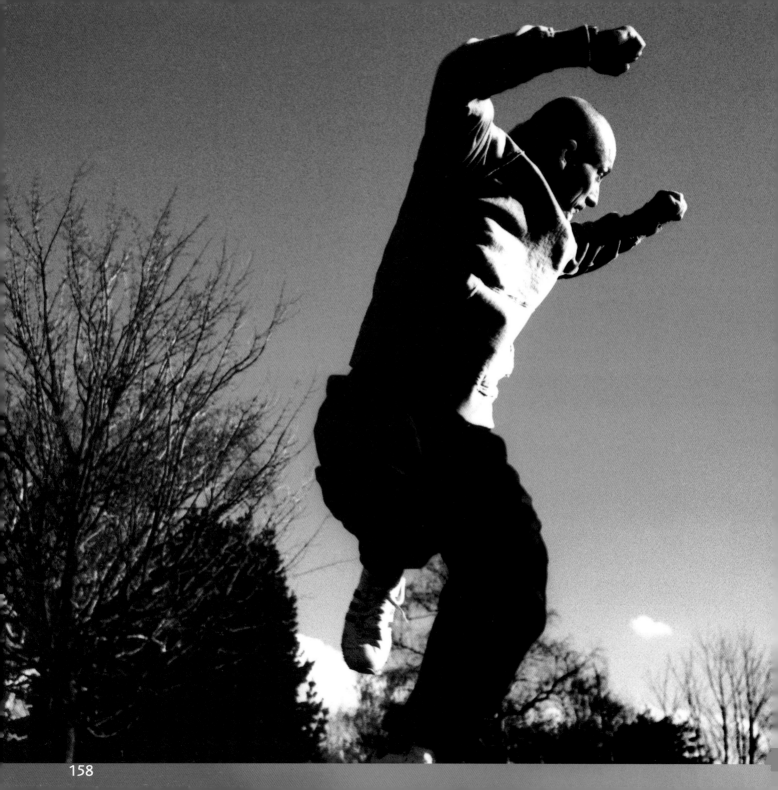

CHAPTER 3
Energy plans

Having looked at what energy is, why we need it, and how to increase it, let's now turn to some energy plans, specially designed to maximize your energy using many of the tools (therapies, diet, exercise) discussed in the first two chapters. So, without further ado, let's turn the theory into practice.

When doing any of the energy plans in this chapter, it is a good idea to keep a diary of how you feel. Begin the diary a day or two before starting the plan and write down how you feel both physically and emotionally, and anything else that you feel might be relevant. Keep the diary up throughout the plan and after. That way, you can look back and be amazed at your progress.

FOR BLOOD DEFICIENCY

If you are blood-deficient, it is a good idea to include iron, herbs, and brewer's yeast in whichever energy plan you choose; likewise, shiitake and reishi mushrooms are particularly helpful for anyone who is feeling run-down.

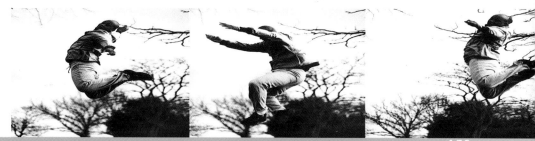

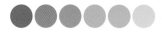
The seven-day energy plan

This plan is specifically designed for anyone who has a heavy week ahead of them or for people who feel that they do have energy, but that they are not functioning at their best. If you lack energy most of the time, one of the longer plans would be more suitable.

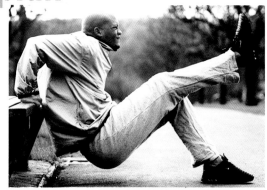

The seven-day plan is designed to provide a maximum energy boost in minimum time, so it is most effective if you can fit in all the elements every day. It consists of core features that you should do every day, with some optional extras to keep you going when you need an extra boost. You will get the best results if you follow the daily routine to the letter. If, however, you miss one or more elements on any one day, don't give up, but do as much as possible of the rest of the plan. You will still be able to feel the difference in your energy levels.

The day before you start the plan, take the time to prepare everything. Plan your meals for the week ahead and go shopping for food, supplements, and essential oils. You will find it much easier to stick to nutritious meals and snacks if you don't have to stop and plan before every mouthful. Set up the oil burner in the position you will be using it or put the oil bottle next to the bathtub, check that you have all the supplements you will be taking, and set the alarm for fifteen minutes earlier than usual if you usually get up and rush out in the morning without eating breakfast.

The daily routine

On rising, drink a glass of hot water and lemon juice to kick start your system.

Do skin-brushing (see page 168) before your shower or bath.

Burn 1–6 drops of invigorating grapefruit oil in a burner, or sprinkle into your bath.

Try to have a thirty-second cold shower after your morning bath or shower. If thirty seconds is just too bracing to begin with, start with ten seconds and build it up day by day.

Do the qi gong slap (see page 112).

For breakfast, choose one of the suggestions on page 165.

Remember to take your supplements.

If you can, do the earth's energy visualization, for example, on the train or bus on the way to work.

Try to fit in a twenty-minute walk—by getting off the train or bus to work a couple of stops earlier than you normally do.

By mid-morning, if you feel your energy flagging, do the standing yoga stretch on page 134.

Don't let yourself get too hungry—eat a snack from the list on page 170 and drink plenty of fresh water.

At lunchtime, have one of the suggested lunches (see page 167). Most of the lunches can be quickly prepared from easily available ingredients and simply assembled at work or at home the night before.

Go for a twenty-minute walk during your lunch break if you haven't done so earlier in the day.

On your way home or when you get home, do the earth's energy visualization if you did not do it in the morning.

If you didn't fit in a twenty-minute walk earlier in the day, go for a walk before dinner.

In the evening, have one of the suggested dinners (see page 171).

Perform the foot massage on yourself, or persuade a partner to do it (see page 57).

Before going to bed, take a warm bath with a few drops of lavender oil sprinkled into it.

In bed or just before going to bed, do the exercise on page 73 to release the tension that has built up during the day.

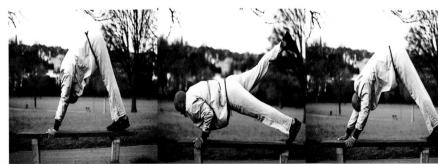

Thirty-four-year-old female filmmaker:

I have been tired ever since I left college about ten years ago. I guess I burned the candle at both ends: I worked very hard and went out a lot; I also had a part-time job, in a club that didn't close till 3 A.M. a couple of nights a week, to help finance me through college. For the last six years I have been making films and still going out a lot. It is a very stressful job, though I do love it and wouldn't change it for the world, but the hours are hard and long, and I often skip meals or eat while filming or very late.

I've tried to do different things to help my energy, like taking ginseng, drinking lots of coffee; I know that isn't good for me, but it gets me through the long days. When it is really busy, I am sometimes so buzzing and full of energy that I can hardly sleep and I feel bad the next day. I realize that this is nervous energy and probably quite bad for me. Some people would probably describe me as always full of (nervous) energy.

Anyway, I decided to do a seven-day plan as I had a big project ahead and had only just finished making a film a few days earlier. I was very tired and worried about being able to get through the next few weeks. I also had a week off, so I thought this would be a good time to do it.

The seven-day plan

Day 1

Am very excited to be starting, but am absolutely shattered. Miss my morning cups of coffee. Forgot to buy the stuff I needed for breakfast, so cheated and had a bowl of sugary cereal. Will go buy food later.

Did the exercises and though I was dreading it, feel pretty good now. Also forgot to buy the vitamins. Ooops!

Day 2

Felt tired still, have started vitamins— feels like a lot to take! Exercised and felt good after. Breakfast felt very healthy— almost forgot to take my vitamins later in the day but have found a little box to carry them in. Wanted wine, but resisted.

If you sit down for a large part of the day, make an effort to take regular breaks—go outside for five minutes of fresh air, walk up and down the stairs, or even just walk around the office to get a glass of water.

SUPPLEMENTS

DAY ONE and DAY TWO

- Vitamin C with bioflavonoids (1,000 mg, once a day)
- Multivitamin and mineral supplement (as directed on the bottle)
- Vitamin B complex (100 mg, three times a day with meals)
- Spirulina/blue-green algae (one pill, three times a day)
- Royal jelly (two capsules, three times a day)
- CoQ10 (60 mg, one with a meal, daily)
- Bee pollen (sprinkle a few granules on food, but stop using if you get a rash or start wheezing, or have any other reactions)

BREAKFAST

- A bowl of fresh fruit, nuts, and sunflower seeds served with natural yogurt
- Oatmeal made with hot water; chop some bananas in and sprinkle some wheat germ on top
- Scrambled/poached eggs with smoked salmon and multigrain toast
- Buckwheat pancakes with applesauce, chopped bananas, and nuts
- Granola with lots of fruit and nuts and skim milk (add sunflower seeds and wheat germ if you like)
- Boiled egg with whole-wheat toast; natural yogurt with seeds, nuts, and fruit on top

Day 3

Still feel tired but not for so long; maybe it is just because I am sleeping more than usual. I do feel more relaxed with the relaxation exercises and I enjoyed the meditation. Went for a long walk today and felt great! Still find the vitamins a bit much but am doing them. Food is good. I thought I would have to eat carrots and mung beans all day!

⬤ Ten-minute sun meditation (see page 78) will provide a quick boost whenever you need it.

LUNCHES

- Feta cheese, watercress, nuts, spinach, and arugula salad
- Broiled chicken sandwich on mixed-seed bread served with a mixed leaf salad
- Avocado, hummus, and alfalfa sprout sandwich on rye bread with salad
- Butterbean and chickpea salad with couscous
- Hummus and tahini and falafel in pita bread with a mixed leaf salad
- Broiled slices of haloumi sheep's cheese with arugula and sun-dried tomato salad sprinkled with sunflower seeds
- Goat's cheese salad with mixed leaves and sun-dried tomatoes
- Beet and kidney bean salad with barley
- Beet, radicchio, and walnut salad with couscous
- Salad of grated celeriac and carrots, with bean sprouts, sprinkled with walnuts
- Tabbouleh made with couscous or quinoa

SUPPLEMENTS

DAY THREE and DAY FOUR
- Vitamin C with bioflavonoids (1,000 mg, twice a day)
- Multivitamin and mineral supplement (as directed on the bottle)
- Vitamin B complex (100 mg, three times a day with meals)
- Spirulina/blue-green algae (two pills, three times a day)
- Royal jelly (two capsules, three times a day)
- CoQ10 (60 mg, two with a meal, daily)
- Bee pollen (sprinkle a few granules on food, but stop using if you get a rash or start wheezing, or any other allergic symptoms)

Day 4

I think I am actually starting to feel pretty good. Am really enjoying the exercises and am going to try and continue when I am working to do some exercises.

Every morning before washing, use a pure bristle brush or loofah to dry-skin brush. Use small circular movements to brush firmly up your arms, legs, and body toward your heart.

EVERY DAY

◉ Drink a glass of hot water and lemon on rising every day.

◉ Try to cut down on caffeine, and if you do reach for it, at least acknowledge that it is a time when you feel tired. If you drink a lot of caffeine, I would not recommend giving it up completely for the seven-day plan because initially, when you withdraw from caffeine, you feel more tired since you no longer have a stimulant pumping around your body.

◉ Drink lots of fresh water.

SUPPLEMENTS

◉ Some people say that they find it hard to remember to take supplements. If this is the case with you, try putting them by your toothbrush for the morning, since you rarely forget to brush your teeth. Alternatively, make it part of your routine to take out your supplements before you sit down to eat.

◉ Many people also feel that they don't like the idea of taking pills at all. If this is the case, you can get multivitamins and B complex in liquid form, and vitamin C, blue-green algae, and spirulina are all available in powder form. Alternatively, some vitamins, such as C and B complex, are relatively easy to find in a food source.

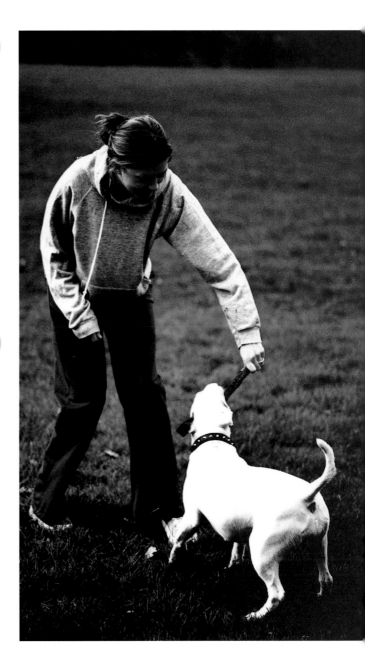

Day 5

Went out and drank a bit last night, so feel a bit worse for wear but still did my exercises and felt better afterward. Regret drinking...I was doing so well...oh, well.

SNACKS AND DRINKS FOR EACH DAY

During the day
- fresh fruit
- assorted bag of nuts and seeds
- bag of dried fruits, especially apricots, figs, and dates
- hummus with carrot and celery sticks
- natural yogurt with seeds, nuts, and fruit on top

DINNERS

- Baked potato with lentil dal
- Stir-fried tofu, vegetables, and pineapple served on a bed of brown rice
- Marinated chicken/tofu/fish kabobs skewered with mushroom, fennel, zucchini, and peppers, served with rice or couscous and a green salad with avocado
- Broiled fish with steamed broccoli and spinach and baked fennel
- Warm grilled chicken salad with roasted sesame seeds and roast parsnips
- Mushroom and feta cheese omelette with Mediterranean vegetables
- Bean burger served with carrot, beet, buckwheat, and raisin salad
- Mushroom pilaf made with brown rice, sprinkled with parsley and cashews
- Squash pilaf made with brown rice, sprinkled with parsley and pine nuts
- Barley risotto with artichoke hearts and feta cheese
- Stir fry of bok choy and shiitake mushrooms sprinkled with cashews

SUPPLEMENTS

DAY FIVE and DAY SIX

- Vitamin C with bioflavonoids (1,000 mg, three times a day)
- Multivitamin and mineral supplement (as directed on the bottle)
- Vitamin B complex (100 mg, three times a day with meals)
- Spirulina/blue-green algae (three pills, three times a day)
- Royal jelly (two capsules, three times a day)
- CoQ10 (60 mg, two with a meal, daily)
- Bee pollen (sprinkle two teaspoons on food, but stop using if you get a rash or start wheezing, or any other allergic symptoms)

Day 6

Back on track again. Feel good. Am in the routine of exercise, good diet, stress relief, etc. Feels great and people are saying that I look a bit "glowing."

DRINKS

- banana and date smoothie sprinkled with wheat germ
- coconut, banana, and pineapple blended with soy milk
- apricot and banana blended with almond milk
- freshly squeezed orange juice
- apple and ginger juice
- peppermint tea

Day 7

It wasn't so difficult. Can't believe it is seven days already! I might continue it for another seven days. I definitely feel like I have more energy and am quite relaxed, too.

ADDITIONAL TREATMENTS

○ Work on acupressure points (see diagram on p. 33) SP6, ST36, LIV3, GB34.

The thirty-day energy plan

This plan is ideal for those people who have energy but would like to improve it or people who normally feel energized but are feeling a bit more tired lately. It is also a good one to do if you know you have a heavy few weeks ahead of you, such as before the holiday season or if your workload is busier at certain times of the year than at others. If you are always tired, the sixty-day plan would be more appropriate for you than this one, but you can always start with this one if the longer plan seems too daunting.

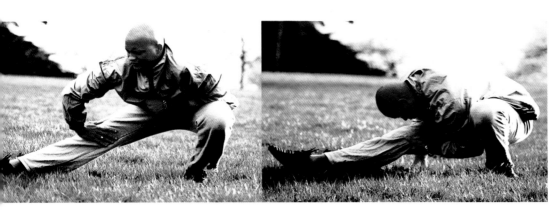

Fifty-year-old businessman

My wife is always telling me I am an overweight couch potato—I think I'm alright although I do feel tired a lot of the time. I only agreed to do the plan because my wife and daughter bet me I'd never get through the whole month.

I nearly didn't make it past the first week—I had headaches and felt really tired, but I had been warned that I might feel like that due to the coffee and sugar withdrawal. So I carried on, but really only to win the bet! I did cheat a bit and didn't follow the plan 100% of the time but I did take the supplements. There's loads of them but I still take them, and I do the exercise, which I love—I'll definitely carry on with the supplements and exercise, if nothing else. I even eat better than I did before (I love cakes and cookies and always used to have coffee and croissants for breakfast).

Everyone says I look great and loads of my friends have started the plan. I've lost weight and I have lots more energy, and I can't believe I don't drink coffee any more!

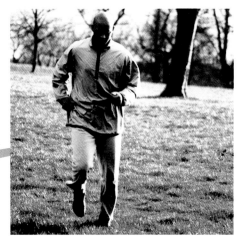

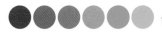
Week 1

Diet

If yours is a typical Western diet that is high in animal protein and fats, refined produce, and additives, and low in fresh, natural plant foods, it would be a good idea to detox (see page 179).

A week's detox program will rid the body of all the residue from the junk food you've consumed. It will also help to reduce your sugar cravings and salt intake, and increase your intake of B vitamins (which will help you to relax) and fiber, which will help the digestive process and speed up the elimination of toxins and waste matter.

You may find that when you start to detox you will feel slightly more tired as the toxins start to come out, but after a week you should feel calmer, more grounded, brighter, clearheaded, and have a little bit more energy. (It takes at least a week, as a lot of toxins lie in the fat tissues.) With a cleaner body, you will have a firm foundation on which to build and really be able to increase your energy.

Eat three meals a day, making them as varied as possible, eating only enough to satisfy your appetite. If you overeat, you will not only build up toxic waste from undigested food, but also become tired from the strain on the digestive system. Drink a quart of water or herbal tea each day, and try to be as relaxed and as calm as possible (relaxation exercises will help).

Diet: examples of daily menus

1. Hot water and lemon on rising in the morning

Breakfast: fresh fruit salad with nuts and seeds; green tea

Lunch: large salad with avocado and lots of nuts and seeds; carrot and apple; ginger juice

Dinner: poached fresh salmon; broccoli and green beans; large portion of brown rice cooked with garlic; chamomile tea

2. Hot water and lemon on rising in the morning

Breakfast: rye bread with mashed banana; green tea

Lunch: lentil and carrot soup; whole-wheat bread; green leafy salad

Dinner: brown rice with roasted vegetables and corn; glass of cranberry juice

3. Hot water and lemon on rising in the morning

Breakfast: half a melon with sunflower seeds; banana and apple smoothie

Lunch: baby spinach, watercress, peppers, tofu, and arugula salad with rice or rye bread

Dinner: lentil and potato pie; green leafy salad with roasted sesame seeds; mint tea

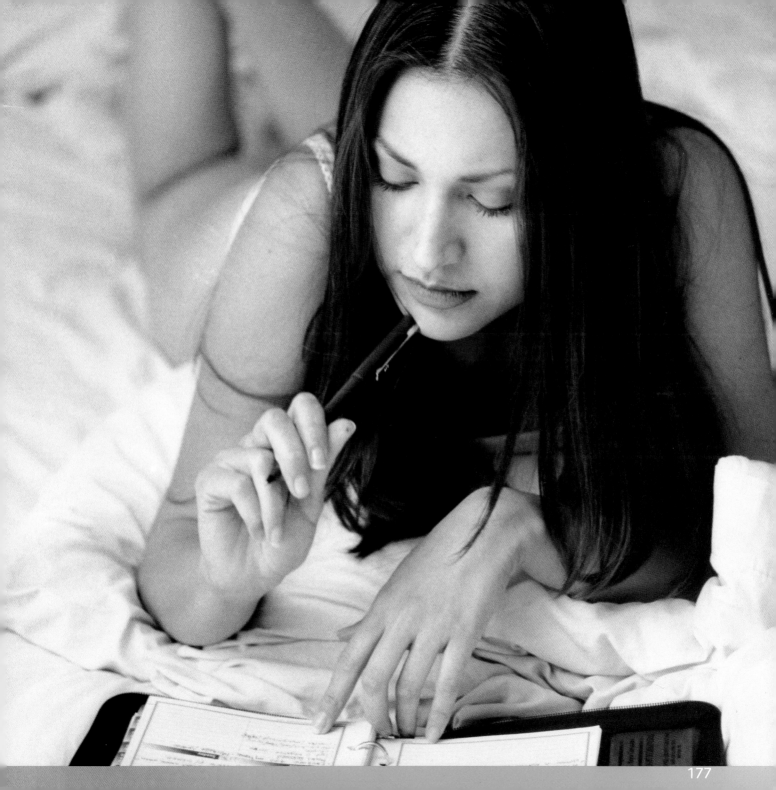

Supplements to start you off on the energy plan:

● See page 179 for supplements to help with detoxification

● Multivitamin and mineral supplement (as directed on the bottle)

● Vitamin-B complex (as directed on the bottle)

Exercise

Every morning, do the windmill (page 104) and the qi gong slap (page 112) or energy sweep (page 117).

Three times a week, do a warm-up exercise, walking, and a cool-down exercise (or at least one other cardio workout).

Try to do yoga postures every day or on the days that you aren't doing cardio. (Remember to do a warm-up exercise before the workout and cool down at the end.)

Energy boosts at work

Do as many of these as you feel you need or can fit into your workday:

● Standing yoga stretch (page 134) and stretch at desk (page 135)

● Relax anytime, anywhere exercise and stressbuster (page 79)

● Ease the tension and private release of tension (page 80)

Self-help/treatments

For this week just do massage with the essential oils to help aid detoxification.

Dry skin brushing (page 168) followed by a cold, invigorating shower for thirty seconds.

Do the posture exercises: standing, sitting, chest stretch, and spinal stretch (pages 136–139).

Do the breathing exercises: alternate nostril breathing and breathing the yoga way (pages 122–123).

Relaxation/visualizations

Every night, do the relaxing the tension before bed routine (page 73).

Do the breath meditation once a day either in the morning, at midday, or when you get back from work (page 76).

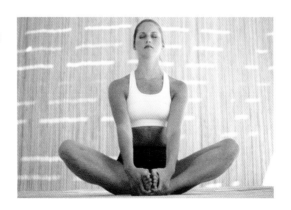

DETOX

Here are some of the dos and don'ts of detox:

Eat lots of: whole grains (especially brown rice), leafy green vegetables, broccoli, peppers, onions, garlic, raw salads, celery, greens, cucumber, herbs, apples, pears, orange-fleshed melon, nuts and seeds (especially walnuts, brazil nuts, and sunflower and pumpkin seeds), pure water herbal drinks, and green tea.

Eat some: fresh fish—but not shellfish (especially mackerel, herring, trout, and tuna), unsmoked organic tofu, olive oil, root vegetables, avocado, bananas, cherries, kiwi, other fruit and vegetable juices, pureed brown lentils, organic pure vinegars.

Avoid: animal foods, dairy products, salt, sugar, refined produce, alcohol, processed foods, high-salt foods, caffeine, nonorganic foods and drink.

NOTE: All foods should be organic and as fresh as possible, eaten lightly cooked or raw.

Supplements to speed up detox

- aloe vera (one capful a day)
- milk thistle tincture/capsules (15 drops, 3 times a day/300 mg a day)
- fresh herbs: dandelion, nettle, parsley, rosemary, and thyme—chop up and make an infusion to drink once or twice a day

Treatments

- Try lymphatic drainage massage by a professional certified practitioner. Lymph massage helps the body get rid of toxins.
- You can also self-massage essential oils into the skin after a bath to help the lymphatic system to work more efficiently (use peppermint, orange, and sandalwood oils in a base oil).
- Brush dry skin to help keep circulation moving and to help the lymphatic system to get rid of toxins, followed by a cold, invigorating shower for thirty seconds.

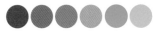

Week 2

Diet

Now that your body is cleaner, you are really ready to start building your energy. The seven-day plan menus are a template for how you should be eating to increase your energy. After trying them, you should be able to create your own meals based on what you have learned so far.

Here's a brief summary:

○ Unlimited fresh fruits and vegetables (not potatoes or sweet potatoes)

○ Lots of water to drink (ideally, around a quart per day)

○ Unlimited herbs, spices, garlic, and vinegar

○ Herbal tea, green tea

○ Natural yogurt

○ Two snacks in between meals—such as unsalted nuts (especially brazil nuts, walnuts, and almonds), seeds (particularly sunflower and pumpkin), fresh fruit (bananas are good), and dried fruit (especially apricots, figs, dates, and prunes), natural yogurt with fresh fruit, cereals

Exercise

Each week, try to do a little more exercise. If you find that what I suggest is too challenging, start slower and build up.

Every morning, do the windmill and the qi gong slap or energy sweep.

Three times a week, do a warm-up exercise followed by at least a twenty-minute walk (or another cardio workout), then finish with a cool-down exercise.

Try to do yoga postures or strengthening exercises every day or at least on the days that you aren't doing cardio workouts (remember to warm up before and cool down after).

Energy boosts at work

As for Week 1

Self-help/treatments

If you need to, continue to practice the postures and breathing until you feel confident that you have mastered them.

○ Practice qi gong exercises: holding the dantien/vital energy (page 110).

○ Repeat affirmations daily, such as: "I can have energy, I want to have energy, I will have energy."

○ Skin brush every morning (page 168) followed by a cold, invigorating shower for thirty seconds.

○ Do shiatsu pressure points SP6, KID1, DU20, LI10, REN4, ST36 (page 33), or beating fatigue and no more blues every other day (page 62)

○ Do your to-do lists (page 82)

2(

Relaxation/visualizations

○ Do the relaxing the tension before bed routine (page 73) every night

○ Do mantra meditation, or continue with breath meditation if you prefer

○ Do earth energy whenever you like, especially if you are feeling very tired

Supplements

When increasing your vitamins, make sure you go slowly and if you have any reactions (loose stools, for example), then decrease the daily intake and increase more slowly.

○ Vitamin C with bioflavonoids (start with 1,000 mg, once a day, and increase to 1,000 mg, three times a day, by the end of the week; continue with this dose for the rest of the plan)

○ Multivitamin and mineral supplement (as directed on the bottle)

○ Vitamin-B complex (100 mg, three times a day with meals)

○ Spirulina/blue-green algae (start with one pill, three times a day, increasing to three pills, three times a day)

○ Royal jelly (two capsules, three times a day)

○ CoQ10 (60 mg—start with one with a meal, daily, and increase to three daily)

Extra:

○ Bee pollen (stop if you get a rash or start wheezing, or if any other allergic symptoms occur)— sprinkle a few granules on your food; if your body reacts well to the bee pollen, you can slowly increase to 2 teaspoons.

○ Wheatgrass (1 teaspoon, once a day)

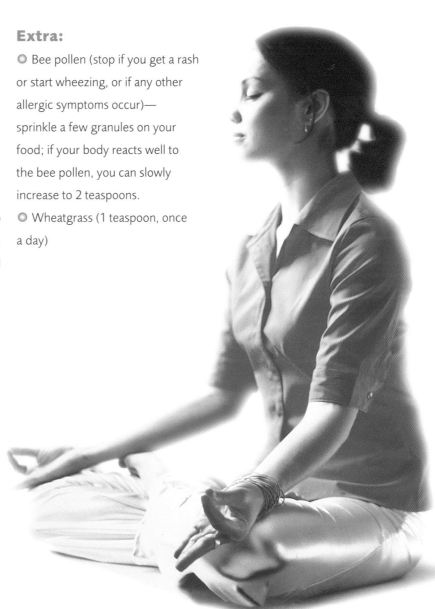

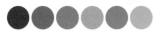

Week 3

Diet

As for Week 2. Try to make your meals as varied and interesting as possible so you don't get bored and stop your new way of eating.

Exercise

As for Week 2 but with more repetitions.

Energy boosts at work

Do as many of these as you feel you need or can fit into your working day:

- Standing yoga stretch and stretch at desk
- Relax anytime, anywhere and stressbuster
- Release the tension and private release of tension
- Walk around the office and take regular breaks from your work/desk.
- Try to get some fresh air.

Self-help/treatments

Practice feeling the energy; you could also do some healing on yourself or on someone else.

Choose some oils to make a blend and either do a self-massage or ask your partner to give you a massage.

Repeat affirmations daily, such as: "I can have energy, I want to have energy, I will have energy."

Skin brush every morning (page 168), followed by a cold, invigorating shower for thirty seconds.

Do your to-do lists.

Relaxation/visualizations

Do the ten-minute sun meditation (page 78) whenever you can or when you feel low in energy.

Do walking meditation or breath or mantra meditation every day (page 76).

Supplements

- Vitamin C with bioflavonoids (see Week 2)
- Multivitamin and mineral supplement (as directed on the bottle)
- Vitamin-B complex (100 mg, three times a day with meals)
- Spirulina/blue-green algae (start with one pill, three times a day, increasing to three pills, three times a day)
- Royal jelly (two capsules, three times a day)
- CoQ10 (60 mg to start with, one with a meal daily, and increase to three, with food)

Extra:

- Bee pollen (stop if you get a rash or start wheezing, or if any other allergic symptoms occur)—sprinkle a few granules on your food; if your body reacts well to the bee pollen, you can slowly increase to 2 teaspoons.
- Wheatgrass (1 teaspoon, once a day)

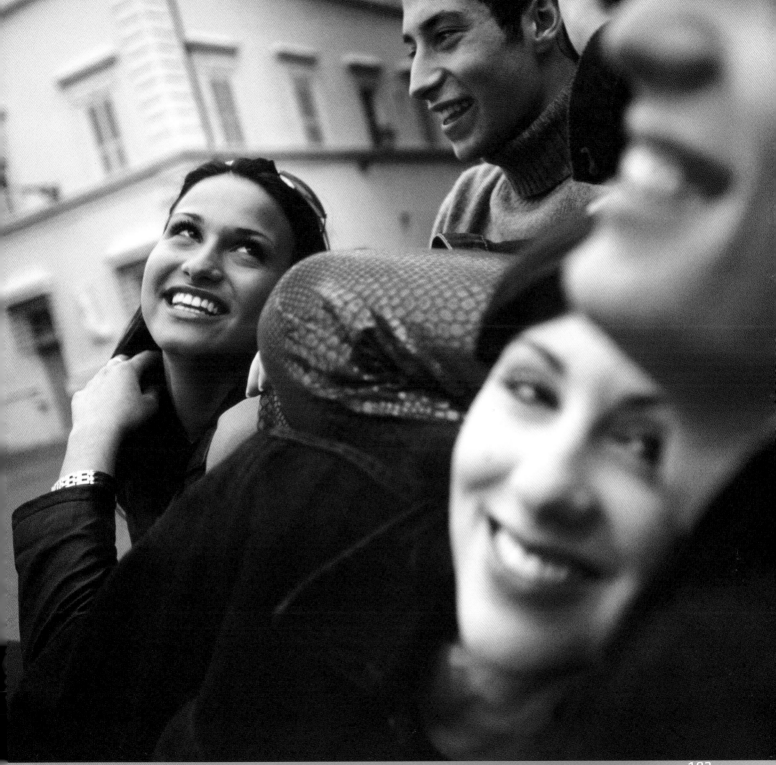

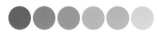

Week 4

Diet

As for Weeks 2 and 3.

Exercise

This week, you are doing your cardio exercises with your strengthening exercises and your yoga.

Every morning, do the windmill (page 104) and the qi gong slap (page 112) or energy sweep (page 118).

Three times a week, do a warm-up and at least a twenty-minute walk (or another cardio exercise), strengthening exercises, and a cool-down.

Do yoga postures every day or at least on the days that you aren't doing cardio exercises (don't forget to warm up and cool down).

Energy boosts at work

Do as many of these as you feel you need or can fit into your working day:

- Relax anytime, anywhere and stressbuster
- Release the tension and private release of tension

Self-help/treatments

Wear bright colors such as red and orange to help make you feel energized.

Make yourself stress tea or revitalizing tea.

Practice affirmations daily, such as: "I can have energy, I want to have energy, I will have energy."

Skin brush every morning (page 168), followed by a cold, invigorating shower for thirty seconds.

Do your to-do lists.

Relaxation/visualizations

Do a meditation twice a day.

Do earth's energy or sun visualization regularly.

Supplements

- Vitamin C with bioflavonoids (see Week 2)
- Multivitamin and mineral supplement (as directed on the bottle)
- Vitamin-B complex (100 mg, three times a day with meals)
- Spirulina/blue-green algae (start with one pill, three times a day, increasing to three pills, three times a day)
- Royal jelly (two capsules, three times a day)
- CoQ10 (60 mg to start with, one with a meal daily, and increase to three, with food)

Extra:

- Bee pollen (stop if you get a rash or start wheezing, or if any other allergic symptoms occur)—sprinkle a few granules on your food; if your body reacts well to the bee pollen, you can slowly increase to 2 teaspoons.
- Wheatgrass (1 teaspoon, once a day)

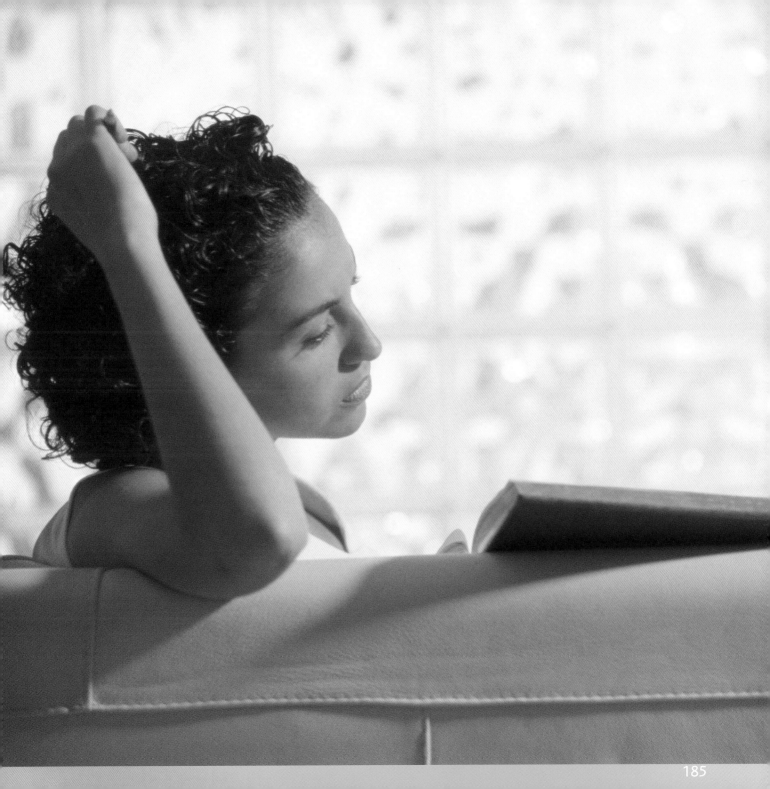

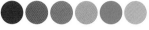
The six-month energy plan

The six-month plan is designed for a person who tends to be tired all the time. It is also good as a maintenance program for people who have enjoyed finding new energy and want to keep up their new energy levels. The idea is to build your strength and energy, and then uphold them. If you stop following the diet and exercise regimes or if you stop taking supplements or practicing relaxation techniques, you will eventually begin to feel sluggish and tired like you used to.

NOTE: If a particular treatment, visualization, or relaxation exercise seems to suit you, don't worry about varying them as I suggest. Just go with whatever is working well for you.

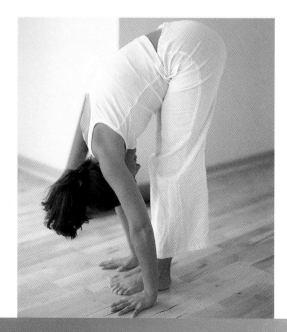

Thirty-three-year-old businesswoman:

I was always tired, which I used to blame on long hours at work, but if I am honest I'd been tired ever since I can remember. I used to get especially tired after lunch and around 3pm. I always needed lots of sleep and was very lethargic, which not only made me feel awful, but also ruined my social life! When Aliza asked me to do the plan I thought I'd never get through it but she told me it would be worth the effort.

The first few weeks were the hardest—I'm not very good at taking pills, exercising, or eating properly, but Aliza told me not to worry and to carry on even if I did slip up every now and then. As for the diet, I always used to be a grab-and-go type person and so I found having to plan my meals difficult. Now I can't imagine why I was worried—I just grab the right snacks instead. Once I got into the swing, it wasn't difficult to carry on for 6 months. I thought it would be harder.

I feel so much more energized and able to go out more—it's embarrassing to admit it, but I can't believe the difference to my social life and my libido!

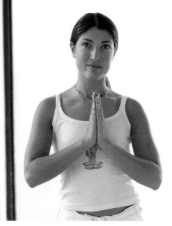

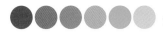
Month 1

Diet

As in the thirty-day plan, begin with a gentle detox for a week and then eat as in the seven-day plan.

Exercise

As for the thirty-day plan, start slowly and then gradually build up the amount of exercise you do.

Energy boosts at work

Do as many of these as you feel you need or can fit into your working day:

- Standing yoga stretch and stretch at desk
- Relax anytime, anywhere and stressbuster
- Release the tension and private release of tension

Delegate at busy times; this will help to get the job done and will also conserve your energy so that the tasks you do are done more efficiently.

Self-help/treatments

Do one of the following at least once a week:

- Diagnose yourself using acupuncture skills, then use acupressure on the appropriate points.
- Visit an acupuncturist.
- Skin brush every morning (page 168), followed by a cold, invigorating shower for thirty seconds.
- Repeat affirmations daily, such as: "I can have energy, I want to have energy, I will have energy."

Relaxation/visualizations

- Do breath meditation every day.
- Do earth's energy whenever you can, especially if you feel tired.

Supplements

- Vitamin C with bioflavonoids (start with 1,000 mg, once a day, and increase to 1,000 mg, three times a day, by the end of first week; continue with this dose for the rest of the plan)
- Multivitamin and mineral supplement (as directed on the bottle)
- Vitamin-B complex (100 mg, three times a day with meals)
- Spirulina/blue-green algae (start with one pill, three times a day, increasing to three pills, three times a day)
- Royal jelly (two capsules, three times a day)
- CoQ10 (60 mg—start with one with a meal daily, and increase to three, with food)

Extra:

- Bee pollen (stop if you get a rash or start wheezing, or if any other allergic symptoms occur)—sprinkle a few granules on your food; if your body reacts well to the bee pollen, you can slowly increase to 2 teaspoons.
- Wheatgrass (1 teaspoon, once a day)

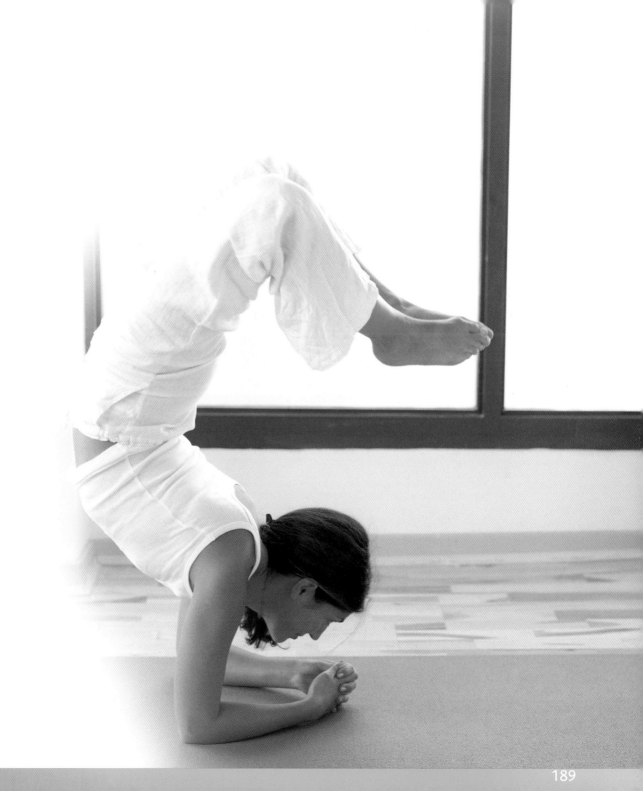

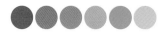

Month 2

Diet

As for Month 1.

Exercise

Make sure you continue to challenge yourself.

Every morning, do the windmill and the qi gong slap or energy sweep.

Three times a week, do a warm-up, a twenty-minute walk or another cardio workout, strengthening exercises, and a cool-down.

Practice yoga postures every day, or at least on the days that you aren't doing a cardio workout.

Energy boosts at work

Do as many of these as you feel you need or can fit into your working day:

- Standing yoga stretch and stretch at desk
- Reax anytime, anywhere and stressbuster
- Release the tension, private release of tension

At home, get others to help with chores.

Self-help/treatments

Choose one of the following to do at least once a week:

- Have an aromatherapy massage.
- Do self-massage using clary sage and lavender oils in an almond base oil.
- Repeat affirmations daily, such as: "I can have energy, I want to have energy, I will have energy."
- Write your to-do lists.
- Do a dry skin brush (page 168), followed by a cold, invigorating shower for thirty seconds.

Relaxation/visualizations

- Do breath meditation twice a day.
- Do earth's energy visualization regularly.

Supplements

- Vitamin C with bioflavonoids (see Month 1)
- Multivitamin and mineral supplement (as directed on the bottle)
- Vitamin-B complex (100 mg, three times a day, with meals)
- Spirulina/blue-green algae (start with one pill, three times a day, increasing to three pills, three times a day)
- Royal jelly (two capsules, three times a day)
- CoQ10 (60 mg, start with one with food daily, and increase to three, with food)

Extra:

- Bee pollen (stop if you get a rash or start wheezing, or if any other allergic symptoms occur)—sprinkle a few granules on your food; if your body reacts well to the bee pollen, you can slowly increase to 2 teaspoons.
- Wheatgrass (1 teaspoon, once a day)

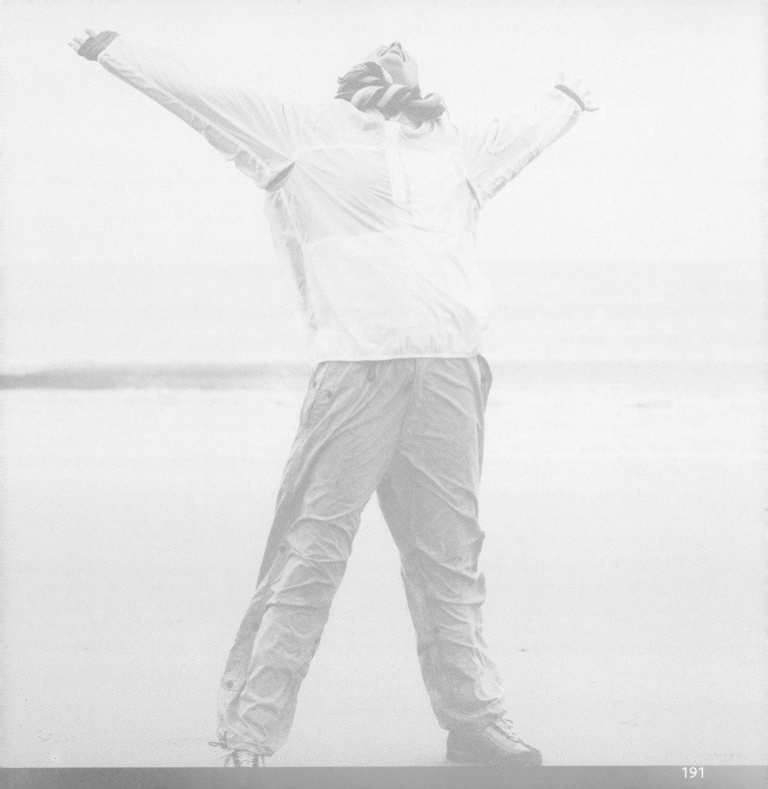

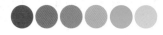

Month 3

Diet

As for Month 1.

Exercise

Every morning do the windmill and the qi gong slap or energy sweep

Three times a week, do a warm-up exercise and at least twenty minutes of cardio and strengthening exercises, followed by cool-down exercises. Do yoga postures every day or at least on the days that you aren't doing cardio (don't forget to warm up and cool down).

Try to walk more often throughout the day; for example, by parking your car farther away or getting off at an earlier bus or train stop.

Energy boosts at work

Do as many of these as you feel you need or can fit into your working day:

- Standing yoga stretch and stretch at desk
- Relax anytime, anywhere and stressbuster
- Release the tension and private release of tension
- Burn basil, peppermint, and/or rosemary in an oil burner to help with mental clarity, or place a few drops on a tissue and inhale regularly.
- Get an ionizer or a salt-crystal light for work.

Self-help/treatments

Do one of the following at least once a week:

- Feel the energy healing exercise (see page 47); then try healing yourself and other people, and get them to heal you (don't try to heal anyone else if you are feeling tired; wait until you have regained all your energy).
- Go to a healer for a treatment.
- Dry skin brush every morning (page 168), followed by a cold, invigorating shower for thirty seconds.
- Repeat affirmations daily, such as: "I can have energy, I want to have energy, I will have energy."
- Write out to-do lists.

Relaxation/visualizations

- Do breath, walking, or mantra meditations twice a day.
- Do shamanic visualization (see p. 150) for increasing energy regularly, especially if you feel tired.

Supplements

- Vitamin C with bioflavonoids (see Month 1)
- Multivitamin and mineral supplement (as directed on the bottle)
- Vitamin-B complex (100 mg, three times a day, with meals)

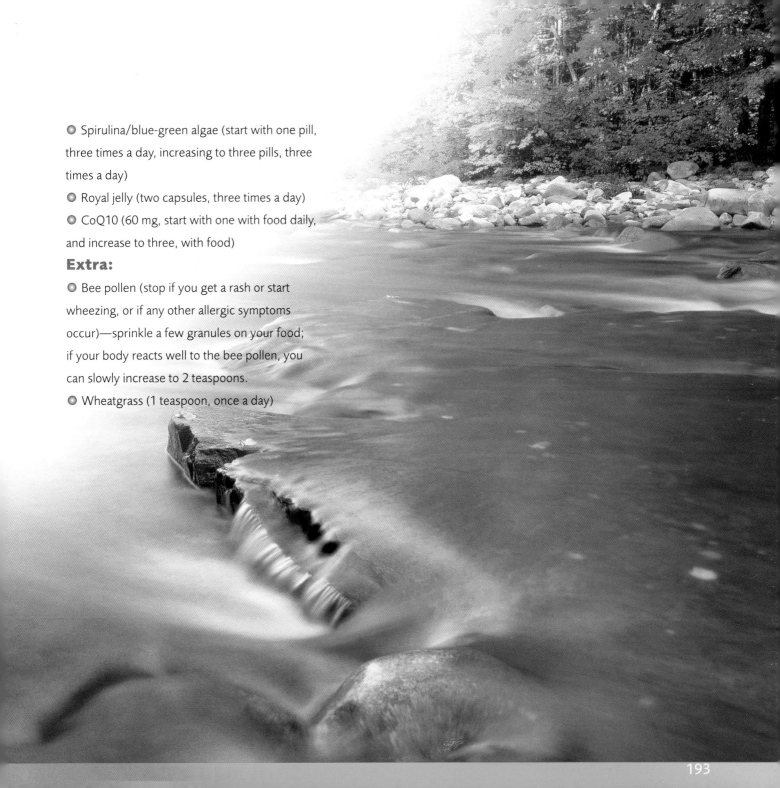

- Spirulina/blue-green algae (start with one pill, three times a day, increasing to three pills, three times a day)
- Royal jelly (two capsules, three times a day)
- CoQ10 (60 mg, start with one with food daily, and increase to three, with food)

Extra:

- Bee pollen (stop if you get a rash or start wheezing, or if any other allergic symptoms occur)—sprinkle a few granules on your food; if your body reacts well to the bee pollen, you can slowly increase to 2 teaspoons.
- Wheatgrass (1 teaspoon, once a day)

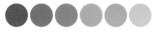

Month 4

Diet

As for Month 1.

Exercise

Every morning do the windmill and the qi gong slap or energy sweep.

Three times a week, do a warm-up exercise, a cardio session (twenty to thirty minutes), and strengthening exercises, followed by cool-down exercises. Practice yoga postures every day, or at least on the days that you aren't doing cardio, remembering to warm up and cool down.

Try to walk everywhere you go and use the stairs isntead of the elevator.

Energy boosts at work

Do as many of these as you feel you need or can fit into your working day:

- Standing yoga stretch and stretch at desk
- Relax anytime, anywhere and stressbuster
- Release the tension and private release of tension

Clean up your desk and throw clutter away. Put a plant or fresh flowers on it, and also hang a quartz crystal on your computer. If there is a window near your desk, open it once in a while for some fresh air.

Self-help/treatments

- Clean your house, one room at a time; throw away things you don't need that create clutter.
- Burn some incense.
- Do some clapping (see page 155).
- Buy some white sage and clean the energy of your home.
- Skin brush every morning (page 168), followed by a cold, invigorating shower for thirty seconds.
- Repeat affirmations daily, such as: "I can have energy, I want to have energy, I will have energy."
- Write out to-do lists.

Relaxation/visualizations

- Do breath, walking, or mantra meditation twice a day.
- Do shamanic visualization or a ten-minute sun meditation regularly, especially if you feel tired.

Supplements

- Vitamin C with bioflavonoids (see Month 1)
- Multivitamin and mineral supplement (as directed on the bottle)
- Vitamin-B complex (100 mg, three times a day, with meals)
- Spirulina/blue-green algae (start with one pill, three times a day, increasing to three pills, three times a day)

- Royal jelly (two capsules, three times a day)
- CoQ10 (60 mg, start with one with food daily, and increase to three, with food)

Extra

- Bee pollen (stop if you get a rash or start wheezing, or if any other allergic symptoms occur)—sprinkle a few granules on your food; if your body reacts well to the bee pollen, you can slowly increase to 2 teaspoons.
- Wheatgrass (1 teaspoon, once a day)

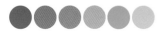
Month 5

Diet

As for Month 1.

Exercise

Every morning, do the windmill and the qi gong slap or energy sweep.

Three times a week, do a warm-up exercise followed by at least thirty to forty minutes of cardio and strengthening exercises, then cool-down exercises. Do yoga postures every day or at least on the days that you aren't doing cardio exercises (remember to warm up before and cool down afterward).

Walk everywhere you go and use the stairs instead of the elevator.

Energy boosts at work

Do as many of these as you feel you need or can fit into your working day:

- Standing yoga stretch and stretch at desk
- Relax anytime, anywhere and stressbuster
- Release the tension and private release of tension
- Buy some wind chimes and put them near a window or wherever you think the energy needs to move or is stagnant.

Self-help/treatments

Do one of the following at least once a week:

- Try to see your aura and other people's auras, and then do the chakra balance (see p. 150).
- Go to see someone who cleans auras and/or balances chakras.
- Skin brush every morning (page 168), followed by a cold, invigorating shower for thirty seconds.
- Repeat affirmations daily, such as: "I can have energy, I want to have energy, I will have energy."
- Write out to-do lists.

Relaxation/visualizations

- Do breath, walking, or mantra meditation three times a day.
- Do earth's energy, Shamanic visualization, or ten-minute sun meditation regularly, especially if you feel tired.

Supplements

- Vitamin C with bioflavonoids (see Month 1)
- Multivitamin and mineral supplement (as directed on the bottle)
- Vitamin-B complex (100 mg, three times a day, with meals)
- Spirulina/blue-green algae (start with one pill, three times a day, increasing to three pills, three times a day)

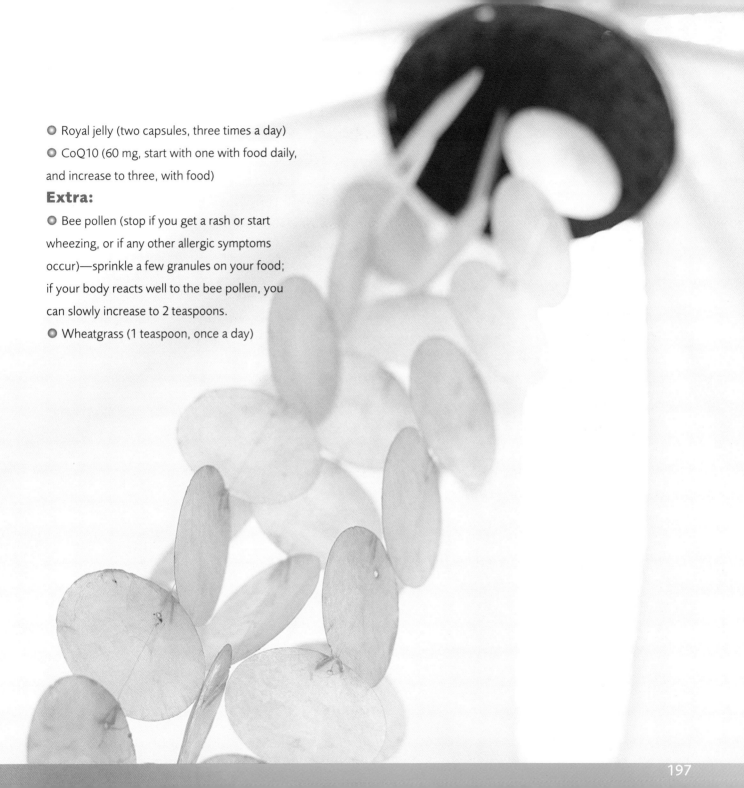

- Royal jelly (two capsules, three times a day)
- CoQ10 (60 mg, start with one with food daily, and increase to three, with food)

Extra:

- Bee pollen (stop if you get a rash or start wheezing, or if any other allergic symptoms occur)—sprinkle a few granules on your food; if your body reacts well to the bee pollen, you can slowly increase to 2 teaspoons.
- Wheatgrass (1 teaspoon, once a day)

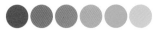

Month 6

Diet

As for Month 1.

Exercise

Every morning, do the windmill and the qi gong slap or energy sweep.

Three times a week, do a warm-up exercise, followed by at least forty to forty-five minutes of cardio and strengthening exercises, and then cool-down exercises. Do yoga postures every day or at least on the days that you aren't doing cardio workouts (remember to warm up before and cool down afterward).

Walk everywhere you go and use the stairs instead of the elevator.

Energy boosts at work

Try to get everyone in your workplace laughing at least once a day; try to look for the funny things in life.

Do as many of these as you feel you need or can fit into your working day:

- Standing yoga stretch and stretch at desk
- Relax anytime, anywhere and stressbuster
- Release the tension and private release of tension

Self-help/treatments

Practice any of the treatments from Chapter 2 that you have enjoyed or have a session with a professional. Try to do at least one session a week.

- Skin brush every morning (page 168), followed by a cold, invigorating shower for thirty seconds.
- Repeat affirmations daily, such as: "I can have energy, I want to have energy, I will have energy."
- Write out to-do lists.

Relaxation/visualizations

- Do breath, walking, or mantra meditation three times a day.
- Do any of the visualizations that you have enjoyed, especially if you feel tired.

Supplements

- Vitamin C with bioflavonoids (see Month 1)
- Multivitamin and mineral supplement (as directed on the bottle)
- Vitamin-B complex (100 mg, three times a day, with meals)
- Spirulina/blue-green algae (start with one pill, three times a day, increasing to three pills, three times a day)
- Royal jelly (two capsules, three times a day)
- CoQ10 (60 mg, start with one with food daily, and increase to three, with food)

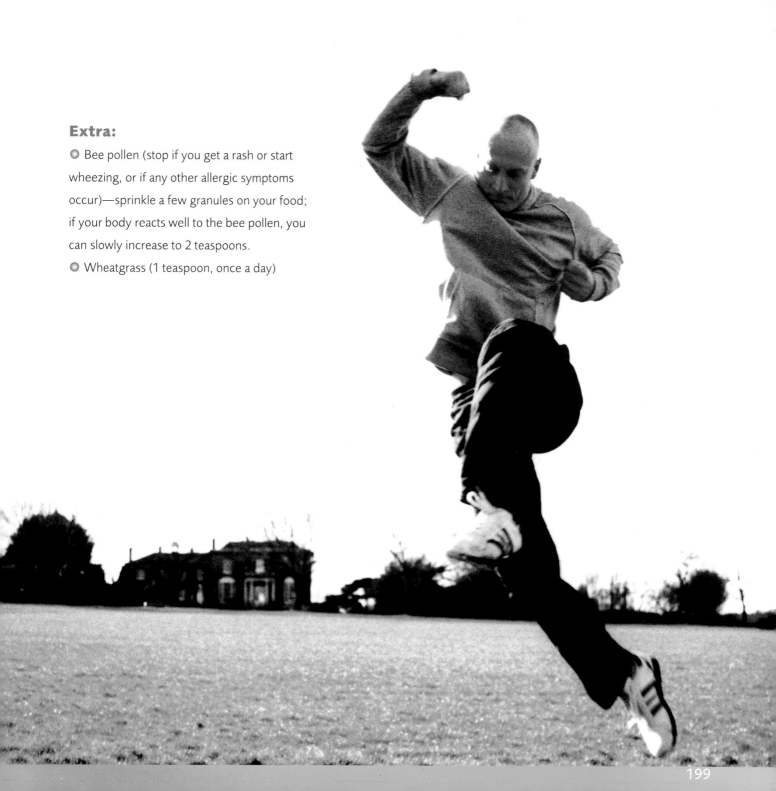

Extra:

◉ Bee pollen (stop if you get a rash or start wheezing, or if any other allergic symptoms occur)—sprinkle a few granules on your food; if your body reacts well to the bee pollen, you can slowly increase to 2 teaspoons.

◉ Wheatgrass (1 teaspoon, once a day)

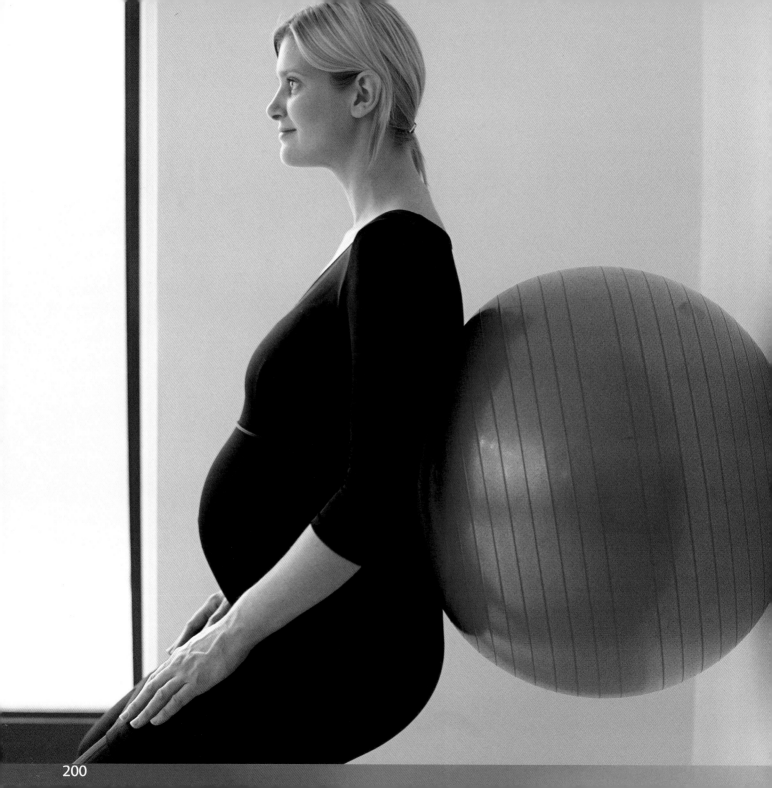

CHAPTER 4
Energy for life

The first few months of pregnancy (the first trimester) are exhausting (I speak from experience, having recently had my first child). The fatigue is caused by physiological and hormonal changes—the hormone progesterone is produced by the placenta and has, among other things, a sedative effect. Hence the fatigue and the propensity to sleep, sleep, and sleep some more!

PREGNANCY

Pregnancy is not the time to start changing your exercise routine to try to increase your energy. The best thing to do is to listen to your body and get plenty of rest. As long as you eat well, rest, and keep a healthy, happy, and positive attitude, you will have as much energy as can be expected.

After the first trimester, your energy will increase, and if you are eating right, exercising, sleeping well, and feeling calm, you should feel full of energy.

Don't undertake any of the energy plans in chapter three when you are pregnant. Instead, go for regular checkups from a qualified physician to help overcome some of the fatigue and other annoying and sometimes unnecessary symptoms associated with pregnancy. Therapies should only be done after the first trimester, and only if they are recommended by your physician. Homeopathy can be good, as well as reflexology and massage.

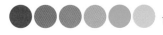

Diet

Eating properly during pregnancy is very important. If your diet is lacking in nutrients, the baby will feed off you, taking the nutrients from your hair, nails, and bones, so you feel even more exhausted and run-down.

All the foods that are recommended for energy are excellent during pregnancy, although it is not recommended to eat anything containing nuts in case of nut allergy in the unborn fetus. Many people believe that a pregnant woman should follow her cravings, as they are often the body's way of telling us what we are lacking. Beware, though, of using pregnancy as an excuse to binge on foods you know are not good for you. Piling on weight will not help you feel energized during pregnancy and will make you feel even more tired when the baby arrives.

Eating regular snacks will help you to keep your energy levels up, and it is important never to miss a meal, which will not only make you feel tired, but your baby will suffer, too. Cutting out caffeine is not only good for the baby, but also helps you maintain your real energy levels.

Only take supplements or herbs during pregnancy on the advice of a fully qualified physician. However, a good prenatal multivitamin and mineral supplement is safe to take. (Make sure it contains folic acid.)

Exercise during pregnancy

A pregnancy yoga class can help ease the stiffness that can often make you feel tired and low. Walking is also good. I found just walking to and from work every day (a twenty-minute walk each way) was a good way to get my circulation moving and supply me with oxygen. I felt great. But always listen to your body, and if you feel tired, stop and rest.

You can also do the exercises for pregnant women (below) every day, since they are very gentle and help keep you slightly active. If you attempt more vigorous exercise, make sure you do so under the guidance of an experienced trainer who knows about exercise during pregnancy. It is often advisable not to start doing exercise during pregnancy if you have never done it before, although gentle walking or swimming should be fine (but consult your physician first). It has been found that women who do some sort of exercise during pregnancy tend to have an easier delivery than those who don't.

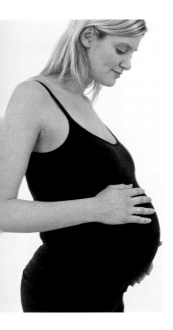

Exercises

Note: Exercise during pregnancy should be done only after the first three months and only after your doctor has given you the go-ahead.

Never strain yourself when exercising, and stop if you feel sick or dizzy.

○ Go for a twenty-minute walk, preferably in a "green" area like a park, to get some fresh air.

1. Kneel on the floor, preferably on an exercise mat, on your hands and knees, with your head in a straight line with your back.

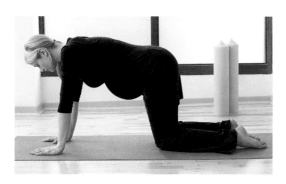

2. Breathe in, then exhale and suck your stomach in (the bigger you get, the more this feels like an exercise!). Hold for a count of five, then breathe in and relax.

3. Repeat ten times.

1. Stand straight, with your right hand supported by a wall or heavy chair/table (make sure that it won't move).

2. Breathe in, then take a step forward with your left leg. Both legs should be slightly bent.

3. Exhale while gently going as low as you can without straining yourself.

4. Breathe in and return to position 1.

5. Now repeat with the right leg, using your left hand to support your body.

6. Repeat five times for each side.

○ Begin cooling-down exercises.

Visualizations and relaxation

Visualizations and relaxation can help with any anxiety you may have about pregnancy and/or the delivery. This is important because anxiety uses up valuable energy that you need for yourself and the baby during the pregnancy, as well as during labor and once the baby has arrived.

Writing a journal can be helpful for recognizing how you are feeling about the pregnancy or how your partner is behaving. It can also be a nice memento to look back on years later.

Many women get surges of energy during the day, and it is important to learn to pace yourself if

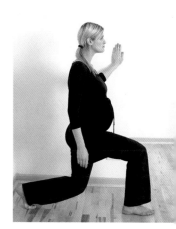

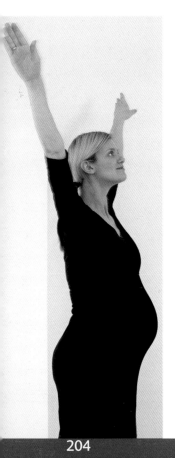

this is the case. It is quite common for women to overdo it during the day and return home in the evening absolutely exhausted. Try to find some time for yourself before the baby arrives, because as soon as she or he is born, your own needs quickly disappear into the background.

As for anxiety before the birth, it is good to try to regularly do some visualizations:

1. Find a time to be alone with the lights low or off and the phone switched off, and get into a comfortable position, either sitting with your feet up or lying on a bed.

2. Try to think about what it is that is worrying you the most, and think of what would you like to happen. If you are worried about the pain of childbirth, then imagine your birth as you would like it to be. Make the picture as clear and bright as possible, and include all the noises you would like to hear (music, for example). Imagine that you are watching a film on a big screen in your head and that you are directing it. It can only be as you want it, so if there is something that you don't like, rewind and rewrite it as you wish.

3. Now that you have decided what you are going to visualize, close your eyes and begin to observe your breathing.

4. Once you are feeling relaxed, start putting your visualization into practice. So, for the example above, imagine yourself going to the hospital as you want it to be, the whole birth, and visualize the beautiful baby waiting to meet you. When you are fully satisfied with the scene you have created, take a mental snapshot, and then when you are ready, open your eyes.

This is a good visualization to do regularly, maybe twice a week or more if you like.

(See also Color Therapy, page 42, for a useful visualization to try during labor.)

Energy for new mothers

Many new mothers say that they feel totally exhausted—because of the lack of sleep, because of the birth (which is tiring in itself), because their hormones are all over the place, and because of their new responsibilities. And that's not even counting all the visits from well-meaning friends and relatives.

It is vital during this trying yet enjoyable time to keep up your energy:

1. Eat healthily. It is often so overwhelming at the beginning that you can't find time to shower or go to the bathroom, let alone sit down to a decent meal. However, it is vital that you eat well and drink lots of water to keep up your strength and energy, especially if you are breast-feeding. (If you are breast-feeding, you must always sit down with a glass of water for yourself when the baby is drinking from you.) All of the guidelines in chapter 2 for eating healthily to give you energy should be followed, but if you are breast-feeding, you can eat more dairy foods and fat than would normally be recommended.

2. Take naps whenever you can. When the baby sleeps, try to take a nap, or at least put your feet up, close your eyes, and relax.

3. Accept help. If you have a friend or family member who is willing to help (and you don't have too many issues with them), try to accept their offers; at first, it might be the only way you are able to find the time for a shower. They might also be able to take the baby for a walk or just baby-sit while you have some time to yourself. It is worth it because you will feel much more energized just for having had the break.

4. Try to stay active. For example, go for walks with your new baby and get some fresh air.

5. It is still important to take your prenatal vitamins (if you are breast-feeding, make sure they are suitable for lactating women).

6. Try to set realistic goals for yourself. For example, try to do one special thing each day, like meeting a friend or going shopping. If you try to do too much, you will exhaust yourself and may feel sad and disheartened.

7. Talk to other people who have recently had babies. It really does help to hear that what you are feeling and thinking is normal. If you spend too much time worrying, you won't enjoy your baby and will eventually worry yourself to exhaustion.

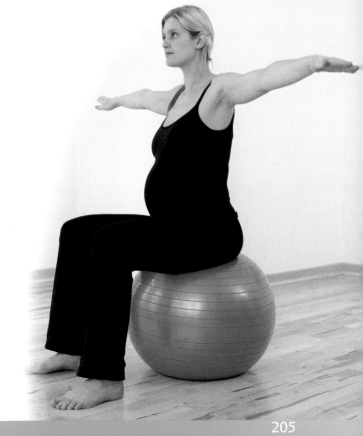

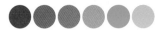

THE OLDER PERSON

Note: Consult your physician before following any of the advice in this section if you suffer from any medical conditions or have any concerns about its suitability.

As we get older, the energy levels of our minds and bodies change dramatically. It does not mean, however, that it's time to retire from life and slump in front of the television just because we are getting older. Concentrate instead on what you can do to strengthen and boost your body/mind connection and your "energy-bank," not just to keep up with life, but to be able to enjoy a good and fulfilling quality of life.

Managing, developing, and maintaining energy as you get older

For a long time, it was commonly believed that the older you get, the more muscle, strength, energy, and vitality you lose. It was said to be an inevitable part of aging. It was also believed that once lost, these things could not be regained or restored. However, this need not be the case, and the stereotype of what it is to look, feel, and be forty, fifty, sixty, or seventy—or older—has changed dramatically from what it was even twenty years ago.

The following have all been proven scientifically:

- Building strength is a great energizer.
- The stronger you are, the easier it is to move.
- Strength lifts depression, giving you the energy to deal with stress—exercise releases endorphins, "feel-good" chemicals in the brain.
- As your internal muscles become stronger, your digestion improves, creating a great feeling

HOURLY APPRAISALS

To maintain energy levels, it is especially important for the older person to do hourly appraisals/check-ins with themselves to become aware if they are overdoing it, while being realistic about what can be achieved.

of leanness in the body and making you feel lighter.

Eating well, exercise, and a positive mental attitude are just as important in the golden years as they ever were before. Regular annual checkups with your physician will enable you to deal promptly with any problem that arises before it starts to slow down your energy.

Plenty of fresh food, fruits, and vegetables should be eaten, along with grains, nuts, seeds, legumes, fish, and plant oils. Calcium, in your food or in supplements, is very important. Avoid smoking and drinking alcohol to excess, and try to maintain a reasonable body weight.

After our twenties, muscle bulk starts to decrease, so it is important to do strengthening exercises; otherwise, muscle loss will lead to strength, stamina, and energy loss, and your metabolism will also slow down. Bone mass can also deteriorate after the mid-thirties, again causing the metabolism to slow down and increasing the risk of fractures and osteoporosis.

Think young

California health writer Deepak Chopra claims you can reverse the signs of aging and regain the body and energy of someone fifteen years your

Controlled experiments were carried out in the 1980s and 1990s, looking at factors that slowed down the aging process and increased energy in the older person. One such experiment looked at people who exercised versus people who didn't. Half of them remained as inactive as they usually were for one year, while the others exercised with weights or did Pilates, isometric, and yoga classes at least twice a week for one year. All of the volunteers were postmenopausal women and not on any hormone treatments. After a year, the inactive group had aged a great deal in terms of muscle, bone, and limb stiffness and weakness. They were substantially less active and less energetic than they had been a year earlier. The women in the group that had exercised were fifteen to twenty years younger in terms of their energy, vitality, and physical condition. They also found that their self-image changed, too. They looked better, felt better, and emotionally they were far more self-confident. It was found that their outlook changed as their inner picture of themselves changed. They were more ready to tackle the full range of challenges that would face older people in the twenty-first century.

junior in just ten weeks. Read on to learn how to turn the emotional and physical clock back by learning new habits, activities, and ways of thinking.

1. Exercise daily. Try walking a little quicker, or park your car farther from your destination than you need to. Swim once a week; walk in the park enjoying the scenery and fresh air. You can even walk briskly around your favorite shopping mall. Do floor exercises once or twice a week.

2. Practice ageless meditation three times a day.

3. Eat foods that are healthy and that you enjoy.

4. Consult a nutritionist, pharmacist, or your doctor for a good multivitamin and mineral supplement to protect against age-related illnesses and find out about supplements for joints and memory, such as glucosamine, chondroitin, and gingko bilboa.

5. Laugh as often as possible! Laughter can help wake up your immune system.

6. Remain curious to keep your mind young, vibrant, and dynamic.

7. Challenge yourself with new experiences, new places, new trends, or new areas of study.

8. Make space for love (not bitterness) in your new life.

9. Stop worrying!

It is important to retrain your mind to feel younger, fitter, and more energized, too. Remember, it is you who will create the new inner picture of yourself and your own idea of the energy you have. Your mind will dictate to your body, and your body will work with your mind. It only takes practice.

Ageless meditation

1. Close your eyes, focus on your breathing, and start to relax.

2. When you are ready, pick an age from your past that you would like to be or that you really feel you are. Make sure you are happy to be this age; if not, choose another age.

3. Repeat the age to yourself over and over, and begin to believe it, feel it; visualize yourself and your energy at that age. Think about how your body feels, what you can do, and your attitudes.

4. Repeat to yourself, "I am a healthy, active, energetic X-year old and I look and feel and act X years old."

5. Once you feel that age and believe you can feel that age, take a mental snapshot that you can take out when you slip back into old patterns or someone says something that makes you feel old.

Repeat this visualization at least three times a day.

VISUALIZATION TO INCREASE ENERGY

To help you "see" your energy and change your inner picture of yourself as an ageless person, try meditation and deep breathing first thing in the morning and last thing at night. Don't be afraid of the word "meditation"—it only means that you are giving your mind and body a small space of time to relax and put aside any stress of the day.

1. Lie on your bed or sit comfortably in a quiet place (you can even do this on an airplane, wearing headphones with the sound turned off).

2. Take five deep breaths and, letting go of all other thoughts that enter your mind, concentrate on the noise of your breathing (in through your nose and out through your mouth). Follow in your mind or "see" the air as you breathe it down the pathway of your spine. Start with the air going down from your neck right down to the base of your spine—that is, the coccyx.

This quiet time will relieve stress, overreactions to situations of all sorts, and help you preserve and maintain the valuable energy you will need both night and day.

Sleep and aging

Many people complain that, as they age, they don't sleep as well as they used to. This is often due to anxiety and stress or poor physical health. Regular activity and more energy will help you be able to sleep better, as has been proven by studies at the Respiratory Sciences and Sleep Disorders Center at the University of Arizona.

Aging with fewer injuries

The more active and flexible you become, the less likely you will be to suffer the recurring injuries often associated with old age. You will also find that if you do suffer an injury, poor health, or have to undergo an operation, you will heal more quickly than you used to if you have managed to remain physically active. Even if you have an injury in one area of your body, you can still exercise other parts to increase your circulation and therefore help promote healing to the affected area. Even gentle exercise will help you recover more quickly from any illness, injury, accident, or operation.

Energy through menopause

Regular exercise will minimize the effects of menopause on your body and mind. Many women who have been exercising regularly up to menopause age do not experience hot flashes or depression.

Even a brisk walk during a lunch hour or dancing to the radio or a CD in the privacy of your own home can help. Exercise can be so effective in the context of menopause that some active women are never really certain whether they have gone through menopause at all. This is because they have no symptoms (besides the telltale sign of losing their periods), and their energy levels remain high, if not higher than they were in childbearing years.

A regular program of exercise provides focus, has a calming effect, and gives energy and a feeling of emotional well-being in menopause just as at other times of one's life.

The correct time to exercise: your own biorhythms for bioenergy

Chronobiology is the study of the relationship between your internal body clock, mood, and behavior. This relationship can affect the biological rhythms that make you feel high (energetic) or low (lazy, sleepy)—the unique patterns inside you that dictate when you should sleep, wake up, do exercise, or have the energy to tackle complex activities.

It has become increasingly accepted by doctors that biorhythms can have a huge influence on your actions, habits, and how you look at yourself. Dr. Michael Hastings, an expert in chronobiology at Cambridge University, claims that "Everything from blood pressure, heart rate, to strength and brain power can change according to the time of day . . . and your genes determine how your body clock works."

Listen to your body clock and how your mind works. Be aware of your energy levels at different times during the day. Maybe you are exercising or doing energetic activity in the morning, but find that this does not suit your mind; restructuring your exercise schedule to keep in tune with your internal clock could help you get the best results.

BENEFITS OF EXERCISE IN OLDER AGE

Studies have shown that exercise can:

- reduce the number of free radicals in your body
- improve cardiovascular health
- prevent diabetes
- increase your energy
- help prevent osteoporosis
- protect against cancer
- help you think more clearly and be able to focus better

Furthermore, according to a study from the University of Illinois, a group of 60 to 75-year-olds who walked at a rapid pace for forty-five minutes three times a week increased their ability to process information and successfully complete tasks. Other research has also shown that aerobic exercise improved high-level brain function in people aged between fifty and seventy-seven. Exercise has also been shown to be as effective as some drugs in treating clinical depression, due to the endorphins (feel-good chemicals) released by the brain during physical activity.

General timings for exercise

- 6 A.M.–noon: Low-impact exercise.
- Noon–2 P.M.: Low-impact exercise, including walking. After lunch, let food be digested, since digestion requires energy.
- 3–6 P.M.: Energetic exercise (adrenaline production is at its highest).
- 6 P.M.–8 P.M.: A good time to swim or do stretching exercises, since the muscles are warm and flexible (adrenaline peaks).
- After 7 P.M.: The body clock is winding down, and you might be disturbing your body clock's natural biorhythms if you demand energetic activity of it at this time; your metabolism will also be slowing down.

Watch your mind and body reactions. Forcing your body to be active when it doesn't want to be will not give you more energy. (Don't mistake this for being out of shape, though.) Just try to tune in to your own body's natural preferences. Then you'll get the most out of your mind and body's natural reserve of energy. Don't be afraid to catch up on your sleep with "catnaps" either, if this is what your body clock and mind dictate; a ten-minute nap will instantly reenergize you. Learn how to make your energy work for you.

What and when you eat should also be taken into account when listening to your body clock. A qualified nutritionist can offer you advice on what to eat, when, and in what quantities to help you reach your most energetic, healthy level of fitness and to help overcome or avoid any complaint or illness. Most feel that you should eat your largest (and heaviest) meal at lunchtime, since your digestive powers are at their peak between noon and 1 P.M. A light supper should then be eaten before 7 P.M., after which time the body needs all its energy for repairing cells and tissues.

Energy for life

The exercises for the older person aim to improve the circulation of oxygen around your body, giving you more energy. They also help combat stress, which is a big energy-robber. Even if you don't feel like doing the exercises to begin with, once you start, you will feel better immediately as you rid yourself of tension. You forget all your problems as you focus on your breathing and the exercise. Also, endorphins are released when you exercise, making you feel happier and full of energy. Try to exercise once a day or once every other day.

Brain training in the "mind gym"

Anyone practicing meditation, visualization, crossword puzzles, or mathematical games is already using the mind gym.

The brain can become stale if you don't challenge it, just as your muscles can become sluggish and stiff when you don't exercise. Try changing your pattern of thinking and acting to alter your mental processes and keep you alert and feeling energetic.

Society's expectations of grandparents (of either sex) and even great-grandparents have grown considerably in recent years. Scientists teach us that our brains can continue to develop throughout life and therefore more is now demanded of older people than ever before.

To help you to keep up with these increasing demands, the "mind tricks" on the next page (based on NLP, or Neuro-Linguistic Programming) can help you change not only how you think, but how you communicate and act, in order to get what you want from life.

TRICKS FOR THE MIND

- Play memory games, bridge, chess, and games that make you think ahead.
- Use the time when you are inactive (such as on a bus or train) but not necessarily relaxing. Don't just sit there—do a crossword puzzle or read a book.
- Change the way that you usually do a routine activity or chore.
- Practice visualizations (such as visualizing a new place or activity).
- Try to make better decisions. Challenge yourself in a new way (make yourself decide things more quickly if you are usually slow, or train yourself to be more careful and thorough if you are usually quick to decide things).
- Focus on detail when walking or meditating. Concentrating on things is a very good mind trick.

Just reading this book is a way of bringing your mind to the mind gym. By reprogramming your memory or altering a belief system, it is possible to change your thought process. The more difficult it is for you to alter your mind map, the more good you are probably doing as far as your brain energy is concerned. A regular challenge should make your brain "sweat," just as your body would if you were exercising.

Stress can cause the brain to function poorly. This may be why yoga and meditation are often practiced twice a day, in the early morning and in the evening, to help the mind counterbalance the stresses of the day and to prepare it to cope with the stresses of the day ahead.

Eating the right foods can help your brain to function. Researchers at Harvard University found that people who only (or predominantly) ate carbohydrates in the morning were less mentally alert than those who ate only protein. Protein provides the amino acids phenylalanine and tyrosine, both of which are needed to produce neurotransmitters, such as noradrenaline, required for concentration.

Give your mind a daily workout and challenge yourself with new and different experiences.

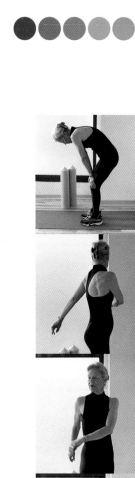

WARM-UP AND COOL-DOWN EXERCISES

Anyone of any age should always warm up and cool down before and after exercise:

⦿ Stand with your feet slightly apart and arms straight.

⦿ Put your hands on your knees.

⦿ Bend your knees and push your bottom out while squeezing it tight. You should be looking down at the floor.

⦿ Repeat ten times.

⦿ Stand with your head up, swing your arms from side to side in front of your body, and look over your right shoulder while your arms swing to the right.

⦿ Repeat twice.

⦿ Stand straight. Put your hands on your ribs and pull/stretch them up as you stand tall.

⦿ Stand tall again, looking at eye level, and roll your right shoulder forward five times and back five times.

⦿ Repeat with the left shoulder.

⦿ Now do both shoulders together five times.

⦿ Kneel on the floor on your hands and knees.

⦿ Make sure that your hands are under your shoulders.

⦿ Look at the floor and make sure that your neck is in line with your back.

⦿ Pull your bottom inward, forming a humpback, then push your bottom back out again so that your back is straight.

⦿ Repeat five times.

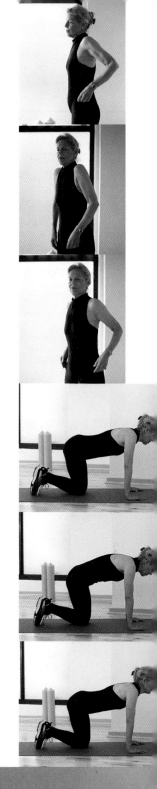

Exercises for people aged between fifty and seventy-five

Always warm up and cool down. Start slowly; build up repetitions gradually.

○ Lie on your stomach with your head on the floor and your hands under your stomach. Push your pubic bone to the floor, breathe in, then exhale and try and lift your stomach off your hands. Breathe in and relax. Repeat ten times.

○ Lift your straight leg up and down (no higher than your hip); keep your bottom tight. Repeat with the other leg. Repeat up to twenty times.

○ Lift both legs off the floor and do little kicks, as if swimming. Keep your bottom tight. Start with twenty and build up to 200 kicks.

○ Mini push-ups: Lift your upper body onto your hands; keep your hands under your shoulders and your hips and legs on the floor. Breathe in and out; raise your back off the floor, extending your arms; lower your body to the floor slowly. Repeat ten to twenty times, building to fifty.

○ Pull your body back so that your chest is resting on your knees and your head is between your outstretched arms.

○ Sit-ups: Lie on your back with your knees up and your feet flat on the floor. Lift your bottom while pulling your back into the floor. With your hands behind your head, lift your head to look at your chest, squeeze your knees together, and breathe in. Exhale and hold the position for a ten count. Repeat ten times, building to twenty.

○ Lie on your side with your legs stretched out in line with your shoulders and hips. Rest your head on your outstretched arm. Rest your top arm straight on your hip; lift your ribs and waist off the floor. Lift both legs off the floor and move your top leg up and down with your foot flexed. Repeat on other side. Repeat ten to twenty times.

○ As above, but this time keep the top leg still and lift the bottom leg up and down to meet the top leg. Repeat ten to twenty times.

○ Roll onto your back, clasp your knees to your chest, and breathe.

Exercises for people aged over seventy

○ The windmill routine (see page 104)

○ The frisbee: Lift up your ribs, stretch back, and stand tall. With your arms straight above your head and palms facing the sky, link your thumbs; with elbows bent a little, move hands and arms like a frisbee, around and around over the top of your head. Repeat five to ten times, changing direction.

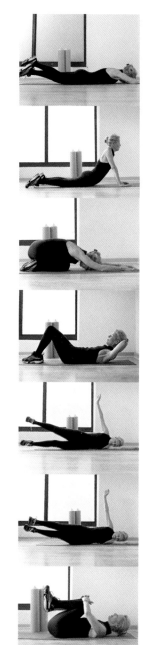

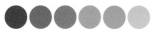 the **energy** plan

Useful addresses

Acupuncture
The American Academy
of Medical Acupuncture
5820 Wilshire Boulevard
Suite 500
Los Angeles, CA 90036
Tel: (213) 937-5514

Northwest Institute of
Acupuncture and Oriental
Medicine
1307 North 45th Street
Seattle, WA 98103
Tel: (206) 633-2419

Allergies
Allergy Research/Nutriology
400 Preda Street
San Leandro, CA 94577-0489
Tel: (800) 782-4274

American Academy of
Environmental Medicine
4510 West 89th Street
Prairie Village, KS 66207
Tel: (913) 642-6062

Human Ecology Action League
P.O. Box 29629
Atlanta, GA 30359-0629
Tel: (404) 248-1898

Aromatherapy
American Aromatherapy
Association
P.O. Box 3679
South Pasadena, CA 91031
Tel: (818) 457-1742

Ayurvedic Medicine
American School of Ayurvedic
Sciences
10025 NE 4th Street
Bellevue, WA 98004
Tel: (206) 453-8022

Ayurvedic Institute
11311 Menaul NE, Suite A
Albuquerque, NM 87112
Tel: (505) 291-9698

Chinese Medicine
Chinese Herbal Medicine
American Botanical Council
P.O. Box 201660
Austin, TX 78720
Tel: (512) 331-8868

American Oriental Medical
Association
433 Front Street
Catasauqua, PA 18032
Tel: (610) 266-1433

Color Therapy
Center for Grief
Recovery/Institute for Creativity
1263 W. Loyola
Chicago, IL 60626
Tel: (773) 274-4600

Counseling
Center for Mind-Body
Medicine
5225 Connecticut Avenue NW
Suite 414
Washington, D.C. 20015
Tel: (202) 966-7338

Feng Shui
Carol Meltzer, BTB,
Feng Shui Master
310 East 46th Street
New York, NY 10017
Tel: (800) 786-5500

Flower Remedies
Ellon USA Inc.
644 Merrick Road
Lynbrook, NY
Tel: (800) 4 BE-CALM
or (516) 593-2206

Healing
The Concord Institute
P.O. Box 82
Concord, MA 01742
Tel: (508) 371-3206

Wellness Referral Network, Inc.
Information and referrals to
doctors and healing arts
providers who focus on
nutrition, illness prevention,
and complementary medicine.
Tel: (800) 520-WELL

Herbalists
American Herbalists Guild
1931 Gaddis Road
Canton, GA 30115
Tel: (770) 751-6021

Northeast Herbal Association
P.O. Box 103
Manchaug, MA 01526-0103

Southwest Herbalist Association
P.O. Box 47
Ojo Caliente, NM 87549

Homeopathy
American Holistic Medical
Association
4101 Lake Boone Trail
Suite 201
Raleigh, NC 27607
Tel: (919) 787-5146

Foundation for Homeopathic
Education and Research
2124 Kittredge Street
Berkeley, CA 94704
Tel: (510) 649-8930

Hypnotherapy
The American Society of
Clinical Hypnosis
2200 East Devon Avenue
Suite 291
Des Plaines, IL 60018
Tel: (708) 297-3317

International Medical and
Dental Hypnotherapy
Association
4110 Edgeland, Suite 800
Royal Oak, MI 48073
Tel: (810) 549-5594
or (800) 257-5457

Martial Arts—T'ai Chi
Patience T'ai Chi Association
P.O. Box 350532
Brooklyn, NY 11235
Tel: (718) 332-3477

Massage
American Massage Therapy
Association
820 Davis Street, Suite 100
Evanston, IL 60201
Tel: (708) 864-0123

Sutherland Institute
4116 Hartwood Drive
Fort Worth, TX 76109
Tel: (817) 735-2498

Trager Institute
33 Millwood
Mill Valley, CA 94941
Tel: (415) 388-2685

Upledger Institute
1211 Prosperity Farms Road
Palm Beach Gardens, FL 33410
Tel: (800) 233-5880

Meditation
American WholeHealth
8150 Leesburg Pike, Suite 700
Vienna, VA 22182
Tel: (703) 827-6567

Transcendental Meditation
Tel: (416) 964-1725
or (888) LEARN-TM

Naturopathy
American Association of
Naturopathic Physicians
P.O. Box 20386
Seattle, WA 98102
Tel: (206) 323-7610

Nutrition
Advanced Nutritional Research
P.O. Box 2639
Mill Valley, CA 94942
Tel: (415) 389-0900
or (800) 569-0444

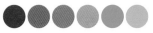
American Diabetic Association
216 West Jackson Boulevard
Suite 800
Chicago, IL 60606-6995
Tel: (800) 877-1600

Biodynamic Farming and
Gardening Association
P.O. Box 550
Kimberton, PA 19442
Tel: (304) 876 2373

Psychotherapy
Psychotherapy Information
Center
59 West 9th Street
New York, NY 10011
Tel: (877) PIC-7939

Reflexology
Laura Norman and Associates
41 Park Avenue, Suite 8A
New York, NY 10016
Tel: (212) 532-4404

Shiatsu
School of Shiatsu and Massage
at Harbin Hot Springs
P.O. Box 889
Middleton, CA 95461
Tel: (707) 987-3801

Stress Management
Stress Reduction Techniques
The Academy for Guided
Imagery
P.O. Box 2070
Mill Valley, CA 94942
Tel: (415) 389-9324

Yoga
International Association of
Yoga Therapists
109 Hillside Avenue
Mill Valley, CA 94941
Tel: (415) 383-4587

Further reading

Agombar, Fiona, *Beat Fatigue with Yoga*, 2002, Harper Collins

Alexander, Jane, *The Energy Secret*, 2001, Harper Collins

Balch, Phyllis A. and James F. Balch, *Prescriptions for Nutritional Healing: A to Z Guide to Supplements*, 1998, Avery Publishing Group

Baron-Cohen, Aliza and Louisa Walters, Adrian Mercuri, *Blissful Detox: Over 100 Simply Delicious Cleansing Recipes*, 2001, Laurel Glen Publishing

Bradford, Nikki and Sullivan, Karen (Editors), *The Hamlyn Encyclopedia of Complementary Health*, 1996, Hamlyn

Hanley, Jesse L. and Nancy Deville, *Tired of Being Tired*, 2001, Penguin

Karas, Jim, *The Business Plan for the Body*, 2001, Crown Publishing Group

Maxwell-Hudson, Clare, *The Complete Book of Massage*, 1984, Ebury

Mitchell, Emma, *Energy Exercises*, 2000, Duncan Baird Publishers

Murrey, Michael and Joseph E. Pizzorno, *The Encyclopedia of Natural Medicine*, 1998, Little, Brown

Van Straten, Michael and Barbara Griggs, *Superfoods*, 2000, Lothian Publishing

Westwood, Christine, *Aromatherapy: A Guide for Home Use*, 1991, Amberwood Publishing

White, Ian, *Australian Bush Flower Essences*, 1993, Findhorn Press

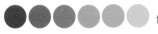

Index

A

acupuncture 6, 13, 16, 30–33
    acupressure points 33, 173
adrenaline 18, 26–27
aerobic exercise 101
aging 206–15
alcohol 11, 18, 84, 89
Alexander technique 136
allergies 22–23, 92
anemia see blood deficiency
aromatherapy 34–37
auras 11, 46, 143–44
Ayurvedic medicine 14, 38–41
    exercise 140–41

B

Bach flower remedies 44–45
balancing diet 87–9
bee pollen 181–82, 184, 188, 190, 192,
    195, 197, 199
blood deficiency 18, 23, 31
    energy plan 159
body awareness 20–21
body clocks 68–70
breakfast 165
breathing 11, 14, 102, 121–23
    alternate nostril breathing 123
    Ayurvedic medicine 39–40
    breathing the yoga way 122
    correct breathing 102
    yoga 121–23
    Bush flower remedies 44–45

C

caffeine 86, 169
candida albicans 23–24
carbohydrates 87
chakras 14, 145–50
    the chakra balance 145
Charles II 35

chest stretch 139
Chinese medicine see TCM
Chopra, Deepak 39, 207
chronic fatigue see ME
clairvoyants 11, 46
clapping 155
cleansing diet 89
clearing 154–55
Cohen, Pete 77
color 143, 146–9, 156–7
color therapy 42–43
conventional medicine 6, 33, 35, 48, 60,
    65
cooking 86
cool-downs 103, 214–15
crystals 46, 67, 142, 144, 155

D

daily routines 161, 169
dehydration 18, 21
depression 18, 25, 66
detox 179
diaries 158, 203
diet 11, 14, 17–18, 68, 84–99
    Ayurvedic medicine 40–41
    blood sugar levels 26, 92
    cultural influences 90–92
    pregnancy 202
    seven-day energy plan 165, 167–68,
    170–71
    TCM (traditional Chinese medicine)
    63–64
    thirty-day energy plan 176, 180,
    182, 184
dinners 171
drinks 170, 172
    water 21, 89, 169
drugs 11, 18
dry-skin brushing 168

E

Earth's energy visualization 78
emotions 18, 58, 67, 151–52
endorphins 32

energy
    assessing 16–17
    boosters 82, 133, 135
    checklist 157
    conserving 9, 83
    definition 11–12
    eating for 85
    enhancers 21
    essential oils 37
    new mothers 204–5
    reserve 17–18
    zappers 18–19, 21
energy plans
    seven-day energy plan 160–73
    six-month energy plan 186–99
    thirty-day energy plan 174–85
essential oils 34–7
exercise 67, 100–9
    aging 207, 211–12, 214–15
    back strengthener 107
    bicep curl 107
    crunch 109
    half push-ups 106
    lateral raise 107
    lunge 108
    pregnancy 202–4
    side crunch 109
    six-month energy plan 188, 190,
    192, 194, 196, 198
    strengthening exercises 106–9
    thirty-day energy plan 178, 180,
    182, 184
    tricep dips 108
    walking 104
    warm-up and cool-down exercises
    103
    windmill routine 105

F

fat 88–9
feng shui 13, 153–57
fiber 89
fitness 21
flower remedies 44–45
fresh air 14, 18, 21, 67

G

Gattefosse, René-Maurice 35

H

Hahnemann, Samuel 48
happiness 13, 152–53
healing 46–47
    feel the energy exercise 47
    healing yourself or someone else 47
health 21, 22–27
    aging 209–10
herbs for energy 65
herbalism 65
Hippocrates 34, 35
homeopathy 48–49, 201
hormone imbalance 25
hourly appraisals 206
hypoglycemia see low blood sugar

I

illness 22–27, 66
immune system 13, 48
ionizers 67, 155

J

jet lag 9, 70

K

ki 11, 13, 61

L

light 14, 154
low blood sugar 26, 92
lunch 167

M

macrobiotics 89–90
mantras, positive 81

massage 50–57, 67, 201
    abdominal massage 57
    aromatherapy 34–37
    face massage 54
    foot massage 57
    giving/receiving massage 50
    head massage 56
    kneading 52
    knuckling 53
    neck massage 56
    self massage 54–57
    shoulder massage 56
    stroking 53
ME (myalgic encephalitis) 24
meditation 11, 74–8
    ageless meditation 208
    breath meditation 76
    mantra meditation 76
    walking meditation 77
mental attitude 81
mental exercise 213
meridians 6, 13, 61
mind tricks for energy 213
minerals 85, 95

N

nadis 14, 145
naturopathy 58
negativity 18, 21, 81, 152–53
nervous energy 19
Neuro-Linguistic Programming (NLP) 77
nutrition see diet

O

overwork 11, 18

P

positivity 21, 81, 152–53
posture 21, 136–39
    chest stretch 139
    sitting 38
    spinal stretch 139
    standing 137

power foods 91
prana 11, 13, 14
pregnancy 8, 33, 35, 48, 60, 62, 64–65, 201–5
protein 87–88

Q

qi 11, 13, 31–32
qi gong 11–12, 110–19
    balancing the energy 114
    energy sweep 118–19
    holding the dantien 110
    qi gong ball 117
    qi gong slap 112
    qi gong tree 116
    vital energy 111
quantum physics 14
quwa 11

R

reflexology 59–60, 201
relationships 151–52
relaxation 21, 73–75
    exercises 79–80
    pregnancy 203–4
    six-month energy plan 188, 190, 192, 194, 196, 198
    thirty-day energy plan 178, 181, 182, 184
relaxation exercises 74–80
    ease the tension 80
    private release of tension 80
    relax anytime, anywhere 79
    relaxing the tension before bed 73
stressbuster 79
    rituals 11, 155

S

sedentary lifestyle 18, 165
self-help
    six-month energy plan 188, 190, 192, 194, 196, 198
    thirty-day energy plan 178, 180, 182, 184

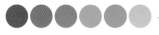

self-massage 54-57
seven-day energy plan 160–73
shamans 11, 150
    shamanic visualization for increasing
    energy 150
shiatsu 61–62
    beating fatigue 62
    no more blues 62
sitting 138
six-month energy plan 186–99
sleep 13–14, 17–18, 21, 66–73
    aging 209
sleeping pills 18
smoking 11, 18, 58
smudging 155
snacks 170
Socrates 48
space clearing 154–55
    clapping 155
    clearing rituals 155
    smudging 155
spinal stretch 139
spine 14
standing 137
stimulants 18–19, 84, 86
strengthening exercises 106–9
stress 9, 11–12, 18–19, 26–27, 58, 66,
    71–73
stretches 134, 139
    stretch at your desk 135
structured time 82–83
Sun meditation 78
supplements 93–97, 165, 167, 169, 171
    seven-day energy plan 167, 169,
    171
    six-month energy plan 188, 190,
    192–98
    thirty-day energy plan 178, 181,
    182, 184

T

t'ai chi 11
TCM (Traditional Chinese Medicine) 6,
    13, 63–64
therapists 29
thirty-day energy plan 174–85
tiredness 8–9, 17, 22–27
to-do lists 82–83
travel 9, 90, 109

V

Valnet, Dr. 35
vibrational energy 142–57
visualizations 77–88, 150
    aging 209
    Earth's energy visualization 78
    pregnancy visualizations 42, 209
    shamanic visualization for increasing
    energy 150
    six-month energy plan 188, 190,
    192, 194, 196, 198
    ten-minute sun visualization 78
    thirty-day energy plan 178, 181–82,
    184
    visualization to increase energy 209
vitamins 85, 93–95
    in food 94–95

W

walking 77, 104
warm-ups 103, 214–15
wheatgrass 181–82, 184, 188, 190, 192,
    195, 197, 199
windmill routine 104–5, 215
work 82–83, 133, 135
    six-month energy plan 188, 190,
    192, 194, 196, 198
    thirty-day energy plan 178, 180,
    182, 184

Y

yoga 11–12, 14, 120–35
    alternate nostril breathing 123
    backward stretch 131
    the bow 132
    breathing the yoga way 122
    the bridge 129
    the butterfly 131
    energy triangle 127
    exercises 124–32, 134
    the fish 129
    forward stretch 131
    half shoulder stand 128
    hand clasp 130
    head-to-knee pose 128
    leg raises 128
    the lion 130
    pose of a child 132
    sitting lotus 124
    standing yoga stretch 134
    sun salutation 125–26

Publisher's acknowledgments

The publisher would like to thank the following for their kind permission to reproduce the images on the following pages.

1, 2–3 Getty Images; **6–7** Photonica/Cheryl Koralik; **8** Photonica/ Cheryl Koralik; **9** Photonica/Mia Klein; **10** Photonica/Mitsuru Yamaguchi; **12** Photonica/Nicholas Pavloff; **13** Getty Images; **15** Bubbles; **16** Getty Images; **18** Francesca York; **19** Powerstock **23** Getty Images; **24** Photonica/Niki Sianni; **25** Photonica/Jen Fong; **26** Getty Images; **27** Powerstock; **28** robertharding.com; **29** robertharding.com; **30** Ray Main/Mainstream; **31** Getty Images; **37** Getty Images; **41** Getty Images; **44** Clay Perry; **45** Clay Perry; **46** Photonica/Kerama; **49** Getty Images; **58** Photonica/Tulla Booth; **66** Getty Images; **67** Photonica/Neo Vision; **68** Getty Images; **70** Ray Main/Mainstream; **72** Bubbles; **88** Getty Images; **140** (running) robertharding.com, (basketball) Powerstock; **141** Powerstock; **142** Getty Images; **150** Getty Images; **151** Getty Images; **152** Bubbles; **155** Getty Images; **156** Photonica/Johner; **157** Photonica/Lisa Stancati; **177** Photonica/ Paul Vozdic; **178** Getty Images; **181** Getty Images; **183** Getty Images; **185** Getty Images; **191** Getty Images; **193** Powerstock; **197** Ray Main/Mainstream; **208** Photonica/ B. Schmid; **212** Photonica/Brigit Utech

The publisher would also like to thank Casalls (c/o Viva (U.K.) Limited, 2 Market Place, Somerton, Somerset, TA11 7LX; England) for kindly loaning the clothes for the photo shoots.

Author's acknowledgments

I'd like to thank my husband Alexis and my daughter Shayna for being so patient with me while I wrote this book. I would also like to thank my mom, Judy (the woman with the most energy and someone I have always aspired to be like), and my good friend Helen, without whom I would not have found the time or space to write. Special thanks to both my friend Lee, who encouraged me to keep going and is always there for me, and to my brother Ash, whose wisdom never ceases to amaze me (although he has never even studied medicine) and who is able to love and support me even though he lives on the other side of the world!

Thanks to all the practitioners at Bliss for their advice and support, and for understanding my absence while I wrote this book. Special thanks to the following practitioners for their expert advice: Deepa (reflexology), Liza (naturopathy), Hari (acupuncture/qi gong), Tara (shiatsu/yoga), Muriel (flower remedies/homeopathy), and Asaf (hypnotherapy). Thanks to Pete Cohen for taking time out of his busy life write the foreword to this book. Thanks also to my mom, my husband, Hari, Tara, Lee, Nathalie, Dodd, and Helen Jones for modeling, especially to those who stood out in the cold with me and my daughter for the sake of a good picture!

Thanks to Helen Woodhall and Kyle Cathie for their patience with my computer failings and also to my dad for sacrificing his own writing to lend me his laptop so I could reach my second deadline!

Last, I could not have written this book without the love and support of my husband—my rock, and the smiles and inspiration of my little ball of energy—my daughter!